W9-BRA-491

Mind
over
Weight

Mind
over
Weight

Curb Cravings, Find Motivation, and
Hit Your Number in 7 Simple Steps

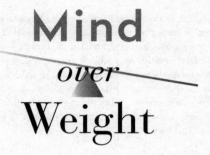

Ian K. Smith, M.D.

ST. MARTIN'S PRESS
New York

First published in the United States by St. Martin's Press, an imprint of St. Martin's Publishing Group

MIND OVER WEIGHT. Copyright © 2020 by Ian K. Smith. All rights reserved. Printed in the United States of America. For information, address St. Martin's Publishing Group, 120 Broadway, New York, NY 10271.

www.stmartins.com

The Library of Congress Cataloging-in-Publication Data is available upon request.

ISBN 978-1-250-24480-2 (hardcover)
ISBN 978-1-250-24481-9 (ebook)

Our books may be purchased in bulk for promotional, educational, or business use. Please contact your local bookseller or the Macmillan Corporate and Premium Sales Department at 1-800-221-7945, extension 5442, or by email at MacmillanSpecialMarkets@macmillan.com.

First Edition: April 2020

10 9 8 7 6 5 4 3 2 1

To my mother, Rena, who has taught me what sacrifice means and how to channel motivation to beat the odds and accomplish goals that others deemed impossible. Your quiet strength has been an endless guide to my life. I will never stop admiring and loving you.

CONTENTS

ACKNOWLEDGMENTS

To Sharon Lieteau, M.D., who shed new light on subjects that would've remained dark for me thanks to her brilliant expertise in psychiatry, generous enthusiasm, willingness to share, and prodigious knowledge of the mind. You are always a cheerleader and great sounding board. I value both and never take either for granted. I love you.

And a big thanks to all of my followers who have asked me for years to write a book about the mental aspects of dieting, and how to find motivation and *keep* it. *Mind over Weight* is in honor of you!

Mind
over
Weight

1

UNLOCK YOUR MOTIVATION

When you think about quitting, think about why you started.

Motivation just might be the holy grail for weight loss and for many other of life's challenging endeavors. Motivation is the X factor, that special ingredient on which the success of the entire recipe stands. You can have the best diet plan ever created, as many trainers as money can buy, private chefs at your beck and call, but if you don't have motivation to start and follow, success will only be a distant pipe dream. Every year, thousands of people purchase diet books and gym memberships, then never once crack the book or cross the turnstile. Without motivation, the best intentions are merely creations of one's imagination. If you want to have at least something of a chance to win the game, then you can't stay on the sidelines wondering what it would be like to get your chance to take a swing.

Motivation is not something that can be gifted, learned, or copied; rather it's something that *must* come from within. Motivation is extremely personal, not something that others can prescribe for you or define for you. Unfortunately, for most people, finding it can seem like an endless search. The truth, however, is that all of us actually possess motivation, but not everyone knows how to unlock it. The mission of this chapter is to help you find and unlock that motivation and understand how to keep it alive and readily accessible. But first let's take a look at the concept of change and its stages that can put you on the road to long-term weight loss success.

In the early 1980s, two well-known researchers, Prochaska and DiClemente, looked at smokers who were able to quit on their own and compared them to smokers who required further treatment. Their study question was quite simple: Why could some quit on their own and others couldn't? The center-piece of their findings was that people quit smoking if they were ready to do so. Given their examination through various studies, the researchers developed something called the Transtheoretical Model (TTM), also referred to as the Stages of Change Model. This is a model of intentional change and focuses on the decision-making of the individual. After all these years, this model is still applicable and widely used

Enter

Precontemplation

Maintenance

Contemplation

Action

Preparation

by therapists helping clients and patients make successful behavioral changes.

The TTM assumes that people don't change behaviors quickly, that change is continuous and occurs in a cyclical process. Studies have shown that people move through a series of stages when modifying their behavior. The original five stages of the model are: precontemplation (not ready), contemplation (getting ready), preparation (ready), action, and maintenance.

✦ **PRECONTEMPLATION.** People in this stage simply are not ready and don't intend to take action in the foreseeable future (usually the next six months). At this point, people are often unaware that their behavior is problematic or can result in negative consequences. They tend to think that others are exaggerating how seriously problematic their behavior is or can be. Precontemplation can seem like reluctance, resistance to being told what to do, resignation to fate by giving up hope that change can occur, or rationalization of behavior. Precontemplators have "all" the answers as to why they don't need to change what they're doing.

✦ **CONTEMPLATION.** People in this stage recognize that their behavior is problematic and that there is hope for change. These people tend to be on the fence. They are open to the possibility of change but aren't completely convinced and haven't made the actual decision to change. There is an intention to change within the next six months, but beyond that, there is no real definition to the commitment. Contemplators are vulnerable to reverting to the precontemplation phase.

✦ **PREPARATION.** This is the stage where things really start to happen. This is the stage of **readiness.** People are committed and intend to take immediate action (typically within the next month). Those in this stage begin to take small steps toward the larger behavior change, and they now truly believe that changing their behavior can lead to a healthier life. All their ambivalence has not been completely resolved, but no longer is it a barrier to change. People will have a plan of action, such as signing up at a gym or purchasing a structured diet plan. When someone is in preparation phase, they are now ready for action-oriented programs.

✦ **ACTION.** This is the stage where people get busy. People have recently changed their behavior (defined as within the last six months) and have serious intentions of continuing to move forward with the change or changes they have made. Those in the midst of action will have shown a modification of their problematic behavior(s) or have begun to acquire healthy new behaviors.

✦ **MAINTENANCE.** People in this stage are pretty far down the road of commitment and action. They have made specific lifestyle changes and are working to prevent a relapse. In the maintenance stage people grow increasingly confident that they can continue to pursue change and not slip back into one of the previous stages.

It's important to identify what stage you're in before starting your program. If you are in the precontemplation phase, it's essential that you are honest with yourself. It's nothing to be ashamed about. It's very normal to say that you want to lose weight, but there can be lots of reasons why you simply aren't ready to do so. The important thing here is that you **don't** start. Trying to start a program when you aren't ready for the change and your motivation isn't where it needs to be will most likely be a futile exercise destined for failure. At the end of this chapter you will have an opportunity to figure out your readiness for change.

Some people spend significant time in the contemplation phase, considering their options and trying to figure things out. Others, however, move through this phase relatively quickly and enter the preparation phase. Many fail in their selected diet program, not because the plan they've picked is ineffective, but because they simply started it at a time when they weren't convinced they could achieve success, or they weren't ready to begin the changes necessary for the plan to work. The process of changing one's lifestyle and behavior requires the alignment of many factors that work in a chain reaction, and the lead domino is timing.

ARE YOU READY TO CHANGE?

One of the most studied and accepted questionnaires for determining readiness for change is the University

of Rhode Island Change Assessment Scale (URICA).
This thirty-two-item self-report measure is simple to
take and can give you substantial insight into where
you fall in the stages of change. I have slightly modified the questionnaire to make it more specific to
our purposes.

KEY: SD = No, Strongly Disagree; D = No, Disagree;
U = Undecided or Unsure; A = Yes, Agree; SA = Yes, Strongly
Agree

QUESTION	SD - 1	D - 2	U - 3	A - 4	SA - 5
1. As far as I'm concerned, I don't have any problems that need changing.					
2. I think I might be ready for some self-improvement.					
3. I am doing something about the problems that had been bothering me.					

QUESTION	SD - 1	D - 2	U - 3	A - 4	SA - 5
4. It might be worthwhile to work on my problem.					
5. I'm not the problem one. It doesn't make sense for me to be here.					
6. It worries me that I slip back on a problem I have already changed, so I am seeking help from others.					
7. I am finally doing some work on my problem.					
8. I've been thinking that I might want to change something about myself.					
9. I have been successful in working on my problem but I'm not sure I can keep up the effort on my own.					

cont.

QUESTION	SD - 1	D - 2	U - 3	A - 4	SA - 5
10. At times my problem is difficult, but I'm working on it.					
11. Seeking help is pretty much a waste of time for me because the problem doesn't have to do with me.					
12. I'm hoping this book or counselor will help me to better understand myself.					
13. I guess I have faults, but there's nothing that I really need to change.					
14. I am really working hard to change.					
15. I have a problem and I really think I should work at it.					

QUESTION	SD - 1	D - 2	U - 3	A - 4	SA - 5
16. I'm not following through with what I had already changed as well as I had hoped, and I'm here to prevent a relapse of the problem.					
17. Even though I'm not always successful in changing, I am at least working on my problem.					
18. I thought that once I had resolved my problem, I would be free of it, but sometimes I still find myself struggling with it.					
19. I wish I had more ideas about how to solve the problem.					
20. I have started working on my problem, but I would like help.					

cont.

QUESTION	SD-1	D-2	U-3	A-4	SA-5
21. Maybe a new program will be able to help me.					
22. I may need a boost right now to help me maintain the changes I've already made.					
23. I may be part of the problem, but I don't really think I am.					
24. I hope that someone here will have some good advice for me.					
25. Anyone can talk about changing; I'm actually doing something about it.					
26. All this talk about psychology is boring. Why can't people just forget about their problems?					

QUESTION	SD - 1	D - 2	U - 3	A - 4	SA - 5
27. I'm seeking professional help to prevent myself from having a relapse of my problem.					
28. It is frustrating, but I feel I might be having a recurrence of a problem I thought I had resolved.					
29. I have worries, but so does the next guy. Why spend time thinking about them?					
30. I am actively working on my problem.					
31. I would rather cope with my faults than try to change them.					
32. After all I have done to try to change my problem, every now and again it comes back to haunt me.					

Scove each statement in the columns below:

PRE-CONTEMPLATION	CONTEMPLATION	PREPARATION (ACTION)	MAINTENANCE
1. _____	2. _____	3. _____	6. _____
5. _____	4. (omit)	7. _____	9. (omit)
11. _____	8. _____	10. _____	16. _____
13. _____	12. _____	14. _____	18. _____
23. _____	15. _____	17. _____	22. _____
26. _____	19. _____	20. (omit)	27. _____
29. _____	21. _____	25. _____	28. _____
31. (omit)	24. _____	30. _____	32. _____

Add the scores in each column. Divide each column's total score by seven to get your average for that column. Add all the averages together to get your total readiness score.

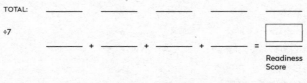

Contemplation + Preparation + Maintenance − Precontemplation = Readiness Score

Scores less than 80 suggest low readiness
Scores above 80 suggest high readiness

MOTIVATION BREAKDOWN

What is motivation? Motivation can be defined as the desire or reason(s) that stimulates, guides, and maintains one's pursuit toward a specific goal or goals. Motivation can be viewed as having three distinct stages:

Stage I: The inner need or drive to do something.
Stage II: A stimulation that arouses this need or drive. For example, you might read a story about someone who overcomes incredible odds.
Stage III: The feeling of satisfaction once the need has been met. You reach your goals and feel a sense of satisfaction.

For the purposes of a weight loss journey, motivation can be broken down into two major categories: intrinsic and extrinsic. Understanding both and their differences is critical to how you find and unlock your motivation, which can help push and carry you along on this transformative journey.

Intrinsic Motivation

Intrinsic motivation centers around behaviors that are driven by internal rewards. The driving force to engage in a particular behavior comes from within the individual because the behavior *itself* brings them satisfaction. Intrinsic motivation occurs without any obvious external rewards. For example, someone reads a thriller written by their favorite author while on vacation, because they love the main character and the types of stories the author weaves. This page-turner is extremely engaging and satisfying. The reader has no extrinsic motivation to read this story, instead they are driven purely by the desire to enjoy the process and experience. This is quintessential intrinsic motivation, and there are several ways to boost it.

✦ **SET CHALLENGING GOALS.** You can become more motivated when the goal you're pursuing has personal meaning that makes you feel strongly about accomplishing it. Goals that stretch your ability but are still attainable can also increase your inner drive. Children who are more advanced than their peers can be demotivated when the teacher is giving them work that's too easy. They don't feel the challenge, so they have less of a drive to diligently complete the assignment or take interest in what comes next. A properly defined challenge that is not too difficult to overcome can be a motivation accelerator.

✦ **BE IN CONTROL.** Having independent control of the goals you choose to pursue can make a difference when it comes to enhancing your internal motivation. When you feel like you have autonomy over your life's direction and your personal environment, you are more likely to be determined to accomplish what you set out to do. Control is empowering, so when you are in charge of deciding what's important and relevant, you feel a greater responsibility and opportunity to achieve what you set out to accomplish.

✦ **ACKNOWLEDGE YOUR EFFORTS.** Be willing to acknowledge to yourself how good you feel about setting your goals and reaching them. If motivation is the fire that makes us burn, self-acknowledgment is the fan that can make us burn brighter. Humility is an important attribute in all that you do and how you carry yourself, but there's no harm in acknowledging truth, especially when that truth is a positive reflection of who you are and what you're accomplishing.

+ **HELP AND COMPETE.** Finding and engaging in situations where you can help someone else can have a positive impact on your intrinsic motivation. There is something about selflessness that fires up the brain's reward-seeking loop and prompts us to make it a priority. Competing can be a tricky scenario when it comes to enhancing motivation, but it's been shown that when you're able to compare your performance favorably to that of others, you are more motivated to continue your efforts.

⇝ **INTRINSIC MOTIVATORS** ⇜

+ Fun/pleasure
+ Satisfaction
+ Gratification

+ Feelings of worthiness
+ Feelings of accomplishment
+ Sense of purpose
+ Pride
+ Developing a mastery

EXTRINSIC MOTIVATION

When motivation arises from outside the person and is driven by the desire for external rewards such as money or fame, it is considered external motivation. It goes back to understanding why you're doing something in the first place. If you're reading a geography book because you want to do well on your geography test, then that is considered to be extrinsic motivation, because the test performance is what's motivating you to study and learn. If you're reading about geography because you simply want to better understand the physical relationship between countries because it interests you, then that's considered to be intrinsic motivation.

One of the advantages of having extrinsic motivation

is that even if the activity or task at hand isn't enjoyable, you're likely to continue to do it because you want the reward that comes with the completion of the task. Homework can often be unpleasurable for students, but they do it because they want a good grade in the class. A musician will practice the same song for hours trying to get all the notes right, not because it's necessarily fun, but because she wants to perform well at her concert.

Extrinsic motivation is used in all kinds of situations, and for many it's just what they need. But this type of motivation can also backfire. It's called the "overjustification effect," and it happens when excessive rewards lead to a decrease in intrinsic motivation. Imagine someone who does a voluntary internship at a veterinary hospital because they want to help care for needy animals. After a few months, the hospital hires the intern to a full-time job and pays him a salary. He is excited that he's now making money and comes to work every day, not because he just wants the satisfaction of helping animals, but because he wants that weekly paycheck that's now allowing him to go out often with his friends. If the hospital suddenly ran into financial hardship and couldn't pay him any longer, would he still come in to help for free as he did as an intern and would he bring the same level of enthusiasm? According to research, it's highly doubtful that he would. Once the overjustification effect occurs, it's very rare for someone to return to intrinsic motivation.

It's the proper balance of intrinsic and extrinsic motivators that seem to form a recipe for motivational success. Do your best to find the combination of those that work for you and put them to work.

⇒ **EXTRINSIC MOTIVATORS** ⇐

+ Fame
+ Praise
+ Grades
+ Money
+ Awards/trophies
+ Social acceptance
+ Material rewards
+ Getting promoted
+ Feelings of superiority

FINDING MOTIVATION AFTER FAILURE

Failure can be the end of the road for desire, but only if you let it. It's not always easy to have great ambitions and hopes only to find them crushed when you don't meet your objectives. It's important that you find your motivation so that you can get back on track and working toward your goals. One of the first things you should do is restate the purpose behind the objectives you're trying to achieve. "I'm trying to lose weight so that my blood sugar levels are lowered and I won't have to go on medications." It's important to remember the "why" when you're trying to figure out the "how." Next, think about the reasons why you failed in the first place. List those reasons carefully, then decide which of those things were in your control and which were out of your control. Focus on those things that you could control, as those are the places where you have an opportunity to do it over again and make improvements. Once you've made this assessment, then it's time to move on and not dwell on your shortcomings.

It's important to look at failure as the spark for

a new beginning, a launching pad that will propel you toward your goals, whether new or old. Adopt a positive mind-set and develop new strategies that will help you accomplish your objectives. Block out the negative thoughts that accompany failure and replace them with thoughts of belief and determination as you make adjustments and accept your missteps as temporary setbacks that you can definitely overcome.

Try these simple exercises to recapture your motivation:

1. **FIND A PLACE THAT AWAKENS YOUR ENTHUSIASM.** Locate an environment that stimulates and motivates you to reach your goals. It might be a hike in the woods or walk along a quiet beach. Find that place that inspires you to go for it, and makes you feel confident that you can achieve what you're setting out to do.

2. **CELEBRATE YOUR SUCCESSES.** Regardless of how big or small, savor and appreciate your victories. When you build on the excitement that comes

with success, you build momentum to keep going and achieve results.

3. **JUST DO IT.** Sometimes our thoughts remain head-locked, and we are unable to advance from thinking about an idea and actually doing it. Stop making excuses, stop overanalyzing, and stop putting it off for the future. Whether it's writing a book you've been contemplating for a while, beginning a fitness routine, or starting a small business, stop thinking about it and just start doing it. Engagement begets more engagement.

4. **ADJUST YOUR FOCUS.** Sometimes what you're focusing on can impact how you feel and your drive to accomplish your goals. How you adjust your focus can be key to how you feel about yourself and what you're trying to achieve. Readjusting your focus can distract you from negative thoughts and clear space in your head to fill with positivity that can inspire you to not give up and continue marching toward your goals.

5. **FIND OTHER VICTORIES.** It's possible to be so engrossed and absorbed in the process of accomplishing something that your energy and creativity can be exhausted. Find victories in areas unrelated to your goals. The excitement of achieving can create momentum that propels you to become engaged and succeed in other tasks you might've lost interest in or felt were too difficult to achieve.

STAYING MOTIVATED

Finding and defining your motivation is half the battle, but the other half is being able to stay motivated. The New Year's weight loss and exercise crush is a prime example of a battle only half won. Millions of people flood the grocery stores and gyms with a new outlook on their health destiny and life in general. They come up with all kinds of reasons why they want to eat better, lose weight, and get more fit. However, several weeks go by and the enthusiasm starts to dim and the motivation starts fading.

According to *U.S. News & World Report*, approximately 80% of resolutions fail by the second week of February. Millions of people who started with good intentions and plans that if followed for the long term would be very effective, quickly find themselves on the sidelines falling back into their old mind-set and behaviors. Why? What changed since they made that serious commitment to do better and adopt a healthier lifestyle? There can be many reasons for this relapse, but a major one is the loss of motivation. So how can you stay motivated and on track? Different strategies work for different people, but here are some that have proven successful for many.

CREATE A REAL PLAN

Part of getting off to a good start is having a good, structured diet and exercise plan to follow. You have the book or the app and you've read what you'll be required to do. Next, it's important to sit down and develop an overall strategy that incorporates your specific goals as well as what you need to get there.

This gives your vision form and helps you better crystallize in your mind and on paper what needs to be done to meet your smaller milestones. Just the process of sitting down and articulating your plans can be a motivator, because your vision moves beyond just a collection of thoughts in your head and is now an actionable plan that's tangible and specific. Once you've completed this larger plan, break it into a weekly plan. This should not be a time-consuming process. Just ten solid minutes and you should have your marching orders written down or typed into your computer or phone. For example, it might look something like this:

WEEK 1

1. Exercise 3 times this week for at least 30 minutes each session.
2. Eat 5 servings of fruits and/or veggies each day.
3. Ride the bike 2 times this week for 2 miles each riding session.
4. Bring a homemade lunch to work at least 3 times.

5. Check in with a weight loss buddy to catch up on things.
6. Replace a solid meal with a shake or smoothie 5 times.

Once you've established a simple game plan for the week, then it's time to quickly break that up into a daily plan. Having specific instructions or goals you need to meet every day in a form that you can see and touch and consult throughout the day can make a big difference in keeping you organized, motivated, and on track. Your daily plan might look something like this:

MONDAY

1. Go to the gym in the morning. Ride the bike for 10 minutes with resistance level of 7. Walk 1 mile on the treadmill at a speed of 3.5 mph, then increase it to 4.0 mph for the second mile.
2. Take a salad with diced chicken to work. Pack a small bag of almonds and 3 cups of air-popped popcorn.

3. Meet up with a friend who works on another floor and take a 10-minute walk at lunch.
4. Purchase two 5-pound dumbbells to use for walks.
5. Do 5 sets of stairwell climbs before dinner.
6. Eat a vegetarian plate for dinner: black beans, broccoli, squash, and carrots.

REDUCE PROCRASTINATION

There is great truth to the adage "Procrastination is the mother of failure." The process of putting things off for another time or finding excuses why you shouldn't begin or complete an action is debilitating and the reason why so many opportunities are missed, and plans fail. Most often, procrastinators find it more difficult to start the task than to complete it once started. You know you need to get up and go to the basement to exercise, but you can't pull yourself out of bed or away from your computer. You keep giving yourself another five minutes, then before you know it, an hour has gone by and then it's time to do something else, and you totally blow the exercise session.

Give yourself the fifteen-minute rule. Set a timer on your watch, alarm clock, or your phone. Once it goes off in fifteen minutes, you *must* get up and begin the task that you need to complete. But before you begin that task, set your timer for another fifteen minutes. Whatever it is you're doing, you can't stop until those fifteen minutes have elapsed. You'll be surprised to find that often when those fifteen minutes are up, you want to continue to perform the task for even longer. And if you don't, the amount you've been able to accomplish in those fifteen minutes may surprise you. We all waste a lot of time avoiding or worrying about things we're putting off rather than plunging right into what we need to do and getting on with it. When you actually get into the groove, your mind-set changes, endorphins—the body's natural happy chemicals—are released, and the task that you thought was too onerous to perform becomes enjoyable and you're motivated to do even a little more than you originally intended.

Sometimes it behooves you to even be early rather

than on time. Not having to rush or feel like you're just making it can be critical to your mental approach to the tasks that lie ahead of you. This can create motivational momentum whereby your head is clear, your intentions are strong, and you get swept up into the feeling that you *can* achieve. You're now excited to do what comes next. The more space you are able to create to work within, the more likely you are to complete what's necessary and not feel the pinch of time. It's no surprise that when a person is rushed, they often don't perform their best, take shortcuts, or simply can't get everything completed. Organizing your time and getting up and being proactive can become self-perpetuating motivation.

SET GOALS WITH ACHIEVABLE MILESTONES

Goals are of no real value if they can't be achieved. Chapter 2 will teach you how to effectively set goals, but it's important to understand that for the purposes of motivation, clearly defined, attainable goals can be a key motivator. It's also important to break these goals into smaller milestones. For example, your overall goal might be to drop your body fat percentage from 25% to 19%. Let's say this might take six to eight weeks to accomplish. It's fine to have that overall number of a 6% drop, but on a weekly basis, you should have smaller milestones that you can hit and feel a sense of accomplishment. A weekly milestone chart might look something like this:

⇒ **TOTAL GOAL: 6% body fat drop** ⇐

START: 25%

END GOAL: 19%

+ Week 1: 1% drop
+ Week 2: 2% drop
+ Week 3: 0% drop
+ Week 4: 1% drop
+ Week 5: 1% drop
+ Week 6: 0% drop
+ Week 7: 0.5% drop
+ Week 8: 0.5% drop

When you can see improvement every week and it's confirmable, that becomes a motivator for you to continue. There is satisfaction that you achieved your goal that week, and this generates excitement and confidence to move on to the next. In some cases, seeing your progress spelled out in front of you might even propel you to surpass your weekly milestone, because a competitiveness is stoked inside you to achieve even more at a faster rate. Sometimes you will miss your incremental milestone. Rather than focus on your disappointment, consider whether it's better to adjust the milestone or identify the reasons why you missed the milestone and make the necessary changes to your strategy or execution of your plan.

REDUCE DISTRACTIONS

It's difficult to stay motivated when your attention is constantly being pulled in all kinds of directions. Cell phones, iPads, computers, social media—so many devices and services are tugging at our senses, time, and energy for most of our waking hours.

We're checking our emails or scrolling through social media right until the moment we close our eyes to go to sleep at night. This sensory overload of being constantly turned on makes it difficult to stay focused and motivated. We spread ourselves too thin and pack our waking hours with so much "other stuff" that we have less time to dedicate to the activities that will keep us on track and making progress toward our goals.

Time is finite, so you have to be wise and judicious in how you use it. Even when you don't think you're being distracted, there are so many things in the background that are working on your subconscious, whether it's a TV, music, or a computer screen with all its blinking lights and scrolling banners. You must be proactive and take action. Every day you should carve out a block of time where you go dark and turn it all off or get away from it all. It might start with just an hour each day, but over the course of several weeks, you might be able to get it up to several hours. This would be a big accomplishment. Once you have taken back control of this time, you can use it constructively to focus on the activities that will bring you closer to reaching your goals or even relieve you of the stress that's blocking your sense of fulfillment and happiness. Streamlining your life and reducing all those superfluous activities and time captivators can open windows of opportunity that you forgot existed or were too distracted to notice.

MEDITATE

When people see the word "meditate," they often think of a dark room with incense burning and soft instrumental music piping in softly from hidden speakers. While this might be a nice environment to practice meditation, by no means is it a requirement. Meditation can take place when you're crammed between bodies in a hot subway car just as it can while you're sitting under a tree in the mountains. Sure, a quiet isolated environment is often more conducive to encouraging and achieving a meditative state, but with practice and focus, the same state can be achieved in that packed subway car.

Meditation is a skill you must learn, just as you

learn to ride a bike or play an instrument. It takes practice and time to truly get the hang of it. It is also a skill that can evolve. Meditation is all about being present in the moment, aligning your physical being with the spiritual. You are trying to get clear perspective on your thoughts, feelings, and your relationship to the world around you. It's not about passing judgment on these things, but rather learning how to understand them.

When you reach that meditative state, you can block out distractions, quiet the chatter not only in the environment but also in your mind. There are different types of meditation, and they are associated with different effects. Here are some of the more common types:

1. **MINDFULNESS.** This is all about being aware and present in the moment. Forget about what's happened in the past or your thoughts or desires for the future. The focus is on the here and now and your existing surroundings. It's critical that you don't make judgments; rather, just make an assessment of the situation.

2. **ZEN.** This form involves specific steps and postures and is often taught by an instructor who has studied the practice extensively. This is similar to mindfulness but requires more discipline, and given the specificity of the steps involved, it can also take longer to learn and more practice. The overall goal is to find a comfortable position that allows you to observe your thoughts without judgment and focus on your breathing.

3. **LOVING-KINDNESS.** The goal of this meditation form is as its name implies—to nourish and cultivate the attitude and spirit of love and kindness toward everything. You are trying to develop feelings where you wish happiness and well-being for everyone—even those who you don't like or have had conflict with in the past.

4. **TRANSCENDENTAL.** This is believed to be one of the simplest and most natural techniques. The goal of this form is to rise or transcend above your current state of being. You repeat a mantra (a usually meaningless sound or series of words) that

commands your attention while your body falls effortlessly into silence.

5. **BODY SCAN.** The goal of this technique is to synchronize the body and mind such that you are totally relaxed and stress is released. Some describe it as imagining a photocopier slowly moving over your body from head to toe and you become aware of all the sensations, discomfort, tightness, and aches that might exist. You learn what you're feeling and where you're feeling it, then release it from your mind and body.

CREATE A VISION BOARD

A vision board is the physical representation of what you envision your success looks like. This is an extremely effective method for keeping your motivation at the top of mind. Take your goals and dreams and find photographic representations of them. You might want to visit the Great Pyramid of Giza one day and cruise the Nile River. You might want to sit atop the Eiffel Tower and have dinner overlooking the lights of Paris. Maybe you want to own a sports car. Maybe there's a dress, suit, or pair of jeans that you want to fit into. Even a beautiful view from atop a hill that you want to be able to climb without getting winded. It might even be a ride at an amusement park that you haven't been able to enjoy because you can't fit into the seat. Whatever your dreams are, find photographs of them, print them out, then pin them to a cork board in your office, tape them to your bedroom closet door, or even post them on your refrigerator with magnets. Vision boards can also be digital. Find pictures and save them in your phone in a vision album, or collect them all in one place on a Pinterest page. Cut out pictures from magazines or newspapers or print them out from the internet and paste them to a vision page in your diary or journal.

Your vision board can also include dreams or goals you've already reached. You could divide your board in half and put pictures of your achievements on one side and what you still hope to accomplish on the other. As you reach your goals, move those items to the other half of the board. The fuller the accomplished side grows, the more motivated you will become to complete more feats and move them across the board.

CREATE A REASONS LIST

Too often we choose to make changes or pursue goals not because it's something we feel passionate about, but because others expect us to do it or we're just following the crowd. It's extremely important to identify and list reasons for why you plan to set out on this journey. These should be your own reasons— not the reasons that others have created for you. There are times in life when it's okay to do something to appease others, but this is not one of them. Your reasons must have important meaning to you, and some of them should connect to the essence of who you are and what you want to be. For true motivation to be effective and sustainable, it must be rooted in truth and authenticity.

Regardless of how great your intentions or how promising the plan you've chosen, doubt will inevitably raise its head at some unexpected turn along your journey. This doesn't make you weak or less well intentioned. It makes you human. Doubt, in some instances, can be a motivator itself. But if you feel like the road is too long or the energy and discipline required of you is too great, then you need something to push you back in the arena. This is why you have that list of reasons. When you are on the verge of quitting, sit down and thoughtfully read the list of why you started in the first place.

≫ ACTION PLAN ≪

1. Take the change assessment to see where you are in your readiness to change.

2. Create your vision board.

3. List 5 reasons why you want to take this journey.

_____

_____

_____

_____

_____

_____

_____

_____

4. Write down 3 things that have motivated you in the past. _____

_____

_____

_____

_____

_____

_____

_____

_____

5. Identify and write down at least 2 intrinsic motivators and 2 extrinsic motivators pushing you to make a
change. _____

_____

_____

_____

_____

_____

_____

_____

6. Write down at least 3 motivational strategies that will
help keep you on track. _____

_____

_____

_____

_____

_____

_____

_____

7. Create 1 or 2 aphorisms that you can repeat. _____

_____

_____

_____

_____

_____

_____

_____

_____

2

THE GENIUS OF
GOAL SETTING

*How successful you are in setting the
right goals is how successful you'll be in
achieving them.*

Setting goals when undergoing personal improvement or transformation is as critical as selecting
the plan itself. In many ways, your goals become
mini-engines that drive you through your plan and
help you overcome the doubts or obstacles or com-
placency that will inevitably set in. In fact, for most
people, goals can also be motivators to stick to the
plan, make good decisions, and stay positive about

being able to achieve ultimate success. Unfortunately, too many people don't take the time to understand how to set appropriate goals, and for many this tends to be their ultimate downfall.

When asked how much they want to lose, some people will say, "I don't know. I'm not counting. I just want to get some extra pounds off me." This approach might work for those who tend to feel overwhelmed by the pressure to establish and strive for a target weight loss goal. But for the vast majority of people, taking this unstructured approach with nonspecific goals can be a fatal mistake. Specific goals are important for many reasons. At the top of the list, goals serve as a gauge of how well you are doing on the plan and indicate whether adjustments need to be made. Adjusting your behavior or the plan itself is critical throughout the process of losing weight, because the variables of weight loss are constantly in flux, and you need to recognize changes and the appropriate way to respond to them. Think about a game of basketball or football. Days before the game, the coaches of Team A devise a game plan on how they intend to play and defeat the opponent.

However, the opponent, Team B, has their own game plan, and they may play in an unexpected way that leaves Team A's game plan ineffective. The Team A coaches will be caught off guard, but that's alright as long as they don't panic and they're able to recognize the ineffectiveness of their original game plan. They must make adjustments to regain the advantage and execute their overall strategy.

On any transformation journey, you must be ready to make the necessary changes to your execution in order to continue your march to success. The tennis icon Billie Jean King simply says, "Champions adjust." If you are going to be a champion on your journey to better health or anything else in life, it's critical that you learn how to recognize when adjustments are needed and how to execute them.

How to Set Your Goals

After establishing that you are actually ready to change, the next step is setting an overall goal of how much weight you want to lose or how many clothing sizes you want to drop. These numbers, however, are just a starting point. Your very next step should be identifying the amount of time you want to take to reach your goal. Let's say you decide you want to lose a total of twenty pounds over a five-month period. Next, break up the total amount of weight loss into smaller goals or incremental milestones so that you can focus on those specific goals right in front of you and not worry about what's much farther down the road. Create incremental milestones by breaking down your large goals and space them out so that as you attain them, you are steadily making progress toward your overall objectives. For example, your twenty-pound weight loss chart might look something like what is shown on the facing page:

WEEKS	POUNDS LOST
1–3	4
4	2
5	1
6	1
7	0
8	2
9–12	3
13	1
14	0
15	1
16	1
17	2
18	0
19	1
20	1

Make sure you also create goals that go beyond the weight loss, for example, exercise at least 3 times a week for 30 minutes each exercise session. You want your goals to be **VERY SMART**—Varied, Effective, Responsible, Yours, Specific, Measurable, Attainable, Relevant, and Time limited.

Varied

Mix up your goals so that you are not focused only on one aspect of your weight loss. Of course, you are primarily concerned about the number reflected on the scale, but there are other parameters that should be on your priority list. How many times during the week are you exercising? How many times during the week are you indulging in fried, fatty foods or overly processed fast foods? Is there a pair of jeans you've been dying to wear, but have been unable to fit into for some time? Maybe you'd like to be able to walk or jog a mile without stopping. Do you want to cut your daily soda consumption in half? There is a long list of goals you can have outside of simply losing weight.

These mini-goals away from the scale are called "non-scale victories" and are extremely important to push you during your overall transformation. Only eating one slice of cake for dessert when you normally have two or walking up a flight of stairs at work instead of taking the elevator are simple examples of victories you can score, off the scale, that can ultimately lead to your success on the scale. Mixing up your goals is important, because it gives you a mental break from always focusing on the number. Too often during the weight loss journey the scale becomes an obsession that can be more prohibitive than it is inspiring. Having a variety of goals allows you to focus on other areas where you can also find success, thus keeping yourself in a positive frame of mind. Maybe you didn't hit your weight loss goal of two pounds this week, but you were able to complete all four scheduled exercise sessions. That is a victory that should be acknowledged and a boost to your confidence that you're still achieving.

Come up with three to five goals that have nothing to do with the scale, and make some of them repeatable goals that you can achieve throughout your transformation journey. Keep track of these goals as diligently as you keep track of your weight loss. Just as you do in the case of your scale goals, make sure you assign some type of reward that's commensurate with what you've achieved.

⇒ NON-SCALE VICTORIES ⇐

+ Hitting an exercise goal (how many times you exercise in a week, distance you walk/run, how intensely you can ride the bike, etc.)
+ Not skipping breakfast for an entire week
+ Not eating a meal within 90 minutes of going to sleep
+ Fitting into a pair of jeans or a dress that's been hanging in your closet
+ Not eating fast food for a week
+ Sticking to your diet plan for 2 weeks without deviating
+ Getting off medication
+ Lowering your blood pressure, blood sugar levels, and/or cholesterol levels
+ Sleeping through the night without waking up
+ Achieving better skin
+ Walking to work instead of driving
+ Walking from the airport security checkpoint all the way to your gate without getting out of breath or breathing hard

EFFECTIVE

Goals should have a purpose and actually produce some type of meaningful change. Let's say you've been diagnosed as borderline diabetic and your doctor says that you need to change your diet, increase your exercise, and lose weight to prevent a full-blown diabetes diagnosis. Then you want to make sure that the goals you set will help you progress to addressing your blood sugar levels. Setting a goal of losing five pounds will not be enough to change your prediabetic status. You need to lose 10% of your body weight, which could be somewhere in the fifteen- to twenty-pound range. So a five-pound goal is not an effective goal and would have no real impact on your outcome.

When you choose your goals, make sure that you are choosing them with the idea that they are going to accomplish something specific. Whether it's increasing your endurance so that you can walk long distances on family vacations or improving your ability to perform yoga positions so that you have better balance, effective goals are the key to reaching long-term success.

Responsible

Goals should allow you to stretch and challenge yourself, but they should also be responsible and not put you in the way of potential harm. Trying to lose weight too fast—for example, twenty pounds in two weeks—can be dangerous if the methods used are extreme and potentially health-threatening. There's no nutritious, healthy plan that I've heard of that can safely help a person lose that much weight in such a short period of time. (The rare exception, of course, is if you're someone who is morbidly obese and have hundreds of pounds to lose. In that case, dramatic weight loss is possible on a healthy weight loss plan.)

Some of your goals should provide a challenge to you, but they should not be so challenging that you need to employ risky methods to attain them. You also have to be respectful of time and make sure that you are not reaching for too much too fast. If you have a goal to run a mile without stopping, and you have never done this before, or it's been years since the last time you've done it, then it wouldn't be wise during the first week of your plan to try to accomplish this goal. Build up to your goal by breaking up the run into smaller continuous segments, slightly increasing the length of these segments every week to ten days, until you actually are able to go the full mile. Setting irresponsible goals often leads to irresponsible behavior or methods, and this is going to impede your success rather than facilitate it.

Yours

Your goals should be just that—*your* goals. You need to own your goals. Setting goals because someone else has said that's what you should do will not work, unless you believe in those goals and take ownership of them. Your significant other or child might want you to lose fifteen pounds because they think you will look better and will be less sluggish. However, if that is not something you want to do or believe in, that is a goal you are unlikely to work hard to achieve. The best intentions of others need to meld with your inner voice if these goals are to be believed in and achieved.

It's easy to get caught up in a competition with others. But setting a goal just to equal or beat a friend or coworker is not a recipe for long-term success. Think about your own goals carefully and what they mean to you and why you really want to achieve them. It's important that your goals have meaning to *you*. Whether it's wanting to look good at your high school or college reunion or wanting to participate in a charity walk, the goal must be one that is important enough to you that you will strive to achieve it. Goal setting is one of the few times where it pays to be selfish. This is all about you, so don't be afraid to have that mind-set when deciding what's most important and possible for you to achieve. However, it's also important to make those in your support group aware of your goals. The better informed they are about your objectives, the better equipped they are to help you and keep you accountable when you are starting to slip or making choices counterproductive to what you're trying to achieve.

SPECIFIC

Most of your goals should be clear and specific so that you can focus your efforts and help stay motivated to achieve the goal. Goals that are not well defined can make you feel like either they're not really achievable or your progress in reaching them becomes difficult to track, so you become complacent and lose your urgency to achieve them. For example, a nonspecific goal would be: "I want to exercise more." The specific and more helpful form of this goal would be: "I want to exercise 35 minutes, 4 days a week, for 3 weeks consecutively." In forming your specific goal, think about the 3 Ws: **what** specifically you want to accomplish; **why** you want to accomplish it; and **when** you want all of this to happen.

⇒ SPECIFICITY IN GOALS ⇐

I want to eat 5 servings of fruit and vegetables 6 days a week for an entire month so that I can reduce my intake of high-calorie fattening food and increase my intake of vitamins, minerals, and other healthy nutrients that will help me lose weight and feel better.

MEASURABLE

Your goals should be measurable. If you're able to measure a goal, then you're able to determine your success in attaining it or how far away you are from reaching it. In some cases (hopefully many), you'll be able to determine how far you've been able to exceed your goal. Being able to measure your goal also can serve as a way to stay motivated and on track. If you know that you have lost eighteen of the twenty pounds you wanted to lose, then you can stay focused on those last two pounds and be encouraged that you are almost at the finish line. Runners who near the finish line after a long run will tell you how they get a second or third wind, an extra boost of adrenaline, even when their legs are tired and lungs feel depleted.

When considering measurable goals, ask yourself three questions: How much? How often? How will I measure the results? If you can answer these questions in your goal, then you've set up something that is concrete, and you'll be able to track your progress to know where you are in the journey. An awareness of your position relative to your goal provides important feedback that can help you modify your behavior or the goal if necessary.

⇉ **MEASURABILITY IN GOALS** ⇇

I want to walk on a treadmill or in my neighborhood 2 miles, 5 times a week. I want to be able to walk these 2 miles in less than 20 minutes.

ATTAINABLE

What good is a goal if you can't attain it? A goal that is out of reach even if you give your best efforts is only going to frustrate you and make you think that you are not doing well, when in reality you are. Unrealistic goals are one of the major reasons why people "think" they have failed at a program or in their transformation efforts. The reality, however, is that they were likely making very good progress, but, because their goal benchmarks were too lofty and unrealistic, they never realize that they were actually making great strides and being successful.

An attainable goal should definitely stretch your abilities, but it must remain within the realm of possibility. Don't set a goal you don't have the resources or ability to achieve. As you are forming your goals, ask yourself how you are going to be able to attain it. Do you have the means and knowledge to reach the goal? Next, ask yourself how realistic this goal is based on any limiting factors that might exist. For example, if you have a lower back injury that limits your mobility, it would be unrealistic to set a goal of doing fifteen burpees in under thirty seconds. While you might want to reach this goal and be willing to work really hard to do so, you physically won't be able to accomplish it. Setting up an unattainable goal is setting yourself up for failure and disappointment.

⇒ ATTAINABLE GOAL ⇐

I own a new blender and I have a freezer full of frozen fruit. Last year, I would make either a smoothie or shake almost every day, but then I got lazy. My goal is to make a smoothie or shake at least 4 times a week and drink it as a solid meal replacement.

RELEVANT

Good goals are those that are relevant to you and wherever you are in your life. It's very productive to have goals line up with other relevant goals so that everything is in sync as it all moves forward together. Good goal setting requires having a focus to your goals so that they make sense in the bigger picture. Let's say your primary goal is to lose thirty pounds in eighteen weeks. This is an important outcome goal. Setting another goal to travel to China to see the Great Wall would not be a relevant goal. It would be fun and adventurous to go see the Great Wall, and by all means, there's nothing wrong with having that on your bucket list of things you want to do, but when setting up your secondary goals that relate to you losing weight, the China trip would not be the most relevant goal. A more relevant goal might be: "I want to be able to walk two miles without needing to stop."

Here are some of the questions you should ask while setting your goals:

1. Does this goal have real significance to my life or other goals?
2. Is this the right time in my life to try to achieve this goal?
3. Does this goal fall in line with or help me achieve the other goals I'm trying to reach?
4. Is this a goal that will help fulfill me?
5. Is this goal worth the work and sacrifice it might take to accomplish it?

PRIMARY GOAL	RELEVANT GOALS
Lose 30 pounds in 18 weeks.	Complete three 30-minute exercise sessions each week.
	Eat only 2 servings of fried foods in a week.
	No white bread or white flour for 2 weeks.
	Bring my lunch to work every other day of the week.

PRIMARY GOAL	RELEVANT GOALS
	No vending machine food purchases for 1 month.
	No eating within 2 hours of going to bed.
	No eating in front of my TV or computer.
	Twice a week, do 2 workouts—one in the morning, one in the evening.

TIME LIMITED

It's important that your goals have some type of time limits connected with them. Setting a goal whose time is open-ended can be demotivating rather than an impetus to keep you focused on making progress. Saying you want to fit into a size 4 dress or lose twenty pounds doesn't have any bite without affixing the time in which you want to accomplish this feat. A specific time parameter is a way to hold your feet to the fire and make you accountable for what you do or don't do to reach a goal. Make a commitment and write it down so that it serves not only as a reminder but a motivator as well. It's much more effective to say, "My goal is to lose twenty pounds in three months." The goal is clear and well defined, and you now fully understand the target you need to hit.

The time limits you set with your goals must also be realistic. Unrealistic expectations are of no value, and in some cases, can discourage you from working to achieve your goal. Let's say you are thirty-five pounds above your preferred weight. The last time you were at your target weight was five years ago. It's unrealistic to then set a goal of losing thirty-five pounds in two months. Is this possible? Yes, but extremely unlikely. Could you do it with the right plan and diligent execution of the plan? Yes, but extremely unlikely. It's unrealistic to expect yourself to achieve such a lofty goal without making dramatic and extreme changes. Be honest and don't set yourself up for disappointment and failure. Give yourself a little cushion in your goal timing so that if you encounter some unexpected obstacles or circumstances, you will have time to adjust and recover. Missing goals can be extremely damaging to the psyche, so avoid being in that position as much as possible to keep your mind-set and motivation undeterred.

REWARD YOURSELF

Setting the right goals in the right away is extremely important in helping deliver weight loss success, but it is only part of the formula. Another significant variable is the presence of continuous motivation that drives you to stick to the plan. We focused on motivation in chapter 1, but it also requires a mention here relative to goal setting. Rewarding yourself for reaching your smaller milestones and larger goals is a proven way to keep you encouraged, determined, happy, and striving to accomplish more.

Building a reward system can be as simple as telling yourself, "When I lose the first five pounds, I'm going to purchase two music downloads that I've been wanting to add to my library." For some people, a simple, largely informal reward plan is all they need to stay motivated and feel like they are accomplishing what they've set out to do. But for many people, it is better to sit down at the beginning of the journey and take fifteen minutes to write down a reward plan that works in conjunction with the goals that you've set up. A well-thought-out and organized reward plan can be a great motivational facilitator, something concrete that you can refer back to often, especially when you are having doubts or looking for something to lift your spirits.

Finding the right rewards and matching them to the right milestones and goals can be an art in and of itself. Making the reward too lofty for a particular milestone can be counterproductive, as the reward's value can surpass the intrinsic value of the milestone reached. If your ultimate goal is to lose thirty pounds in six months, and you divide the goal up to five-pound milestones, then it would be excessive to reward your first five-pound loss with a vacation to Morocco (unless you're a billionaire). Getting a new shiny case for your cell phone would be more commensurate with the achievement, and you would still have the motivation to work harder for loftier rewards that await you further along in your journey.

One reward that I caution against and in some

cases, if it proves to be one of your triggers, outright forbid, is food. It's a good idea to make sure food is not used as a reward or as a punishment, as doing so can further complicate your relationship to food and prompt you, whether consciously or subconsciously, to make unhealthy associations. Instead, choose items or experiences that you've been wanting, but haven't taken the initiative to purchase or do for yourself. Make sure the reward means something to you specifically, whether it's sentimental (printing out an old photograph of you and your friends and framing it), functional (a good blender that is more powerful and easier to use), or fun (a season of a streaming TV show you've been wanting to watch). Make the reward something that is going to make you feel good about your accomplishment, but not so good that you don't want to keep working toward the other rewards that await you.

JOURNEY STAGE	REWARD
Early	2 paid apps for your phone or tablet
	5 music downloads to add to your library
	New case for your cell phone
	Kitchen scale
	Hairstyle change
	Hi-tech or fancy water bottle
	Purchase a streaming season of a TV show
	Pedicure
	New bottle of special lotion or shower gel
	A new plant for your garden
	Purchase a new book
Mid	New blender
	Fun jewelry accessory like a charm bracelet
	One article of midpriced clothing
	Gym membership
	Ticket to a sporting event or concert or comedy show

JOURNEY STAGE	REWARD
	House decoration or furnishing
	New workout clothes
	Small gym equipment for your house
	New bicycle
	Purchase a streaming service subscription
	Sporting equipment like new skis or tennis racket
	Have a professional cleaning service clean your house
	Get a subscription to a magazine
	Take a day off from work and do whatever you want
	A day trip to small town or city you've wanted to visit
Late	Large piece of gym equipment for your house
	Piece of art
	A new purse
	Purchase a new musical instrument

cont.

JOURNEY STAGE	REWARD
	New digital device: phone, TV, tablet, computer
	20 pieces of a new wardrobe
	Trip to a dream destination
	A class: photography, acting, cooking, etc.
	Sit for a professional portrait painting
	Get your furniture reupholstered
	Purchase a high-end camera for vacations

⇞ ACTION PLAN ⇞

1. List your specific goals and milestones. _____

_____

_____

_____

_____

_____

_____

_____

2. Create a detailed goal map.

3. Create 5 goals relevant to your main goal. _____

_____

_____

_____

_____

_____

_____

_____

_____

_____

_____

4. Create a detailed reward system to correspond to your goal map.

_____

_____

_____

_____

5. List 3 non-scale victories you hope to achieve. _____

_____

_____

_____

_____

_____

6. List your most successful past weight loss effort (total pounds lost and time). _____

_____

_____

_____

_____

_____

7. Share your goal map with an accountability partner and task them with helping you stay on track.

3

CHOOSE THE RIGHT PLAN FOR *YOU*

Having goals without the right plan is like building a shiny new airplane and forgetting to attach the wings.

The old adage that there's no such thing as "one diet fits all" is more relevant today than ever. We live in an era of rapid and diffuse information sharing, which stokes the fire for wildly popular dieting trends. Whether it's keto, paleo, or HCG, diets have become as fashionable as haute couture on a Parisian runway. Every few months a new diet bursts on the scene with great fanfare and you can't turn on your television or pick up a magazine without reading about how so many people are dropping pounds on this revolutionary program that's setting the world on fire. While it might be true that these new fad diet programs are helping some of their followers achieve success, the downside is that all the buzz and media attention lead millions to choose programs that simply aren't right for them. So many people test-drive a shiny new plan at the beginning of every diet season, only to find themselves back on a seemingly never-ending diet carousel, because the diet plan proves to be ineffective for long-term success and unsustainable.

There are many reasons why people fail or abandon their weight loss journey, and one that sits on top of the list is choosing a plan that isn't right for them. It doesn't matter what program some Hollywood star followed to lose twenty pounds or what diet took fifteen pounds off your coworker; just because it worked for someone else doesn't mean it's going to work for you. Our bodies are unique, and the way in which we gain and lose weight is also unique. If a program works for others, but doesn't work for you, this doesn't mean it's a bad program. The better way to look at it is that the program simply isn't a good fit for you. A study in the *Journal of the American Medical Association* suggested that it wasn't necessarily the type of plan that was most important when predicting your success in losing weight, but whether you were able to stick to the plan you chose.

So how do you decide which program is best for you when there are so many to choose from and it's so difficult to distinguish one from another? The answer starts with you. Here is your guide for making the best choice.

TALK TO YOUR DOCTOR FIRST

Many doctors don't know a lot about nutritional science, weight loss, and exercise, but talking to a health-care professional is still not a bad place to start. While a doctor might not specialize in weight management, they are still a medically trained scientist who can potentially find the good and bad things in a plan that you might not be able to see. It is particularly important to talk to a health-care professional if you suffer from a chronic illness or you have physical limitations. Maybe you suffer from kidney disease or you have osteoarthritis in your knees or spinal stenosis where a pinched nerve root is causing pain and a lack of mobility. Maybe you are currently being treated for high blood pressure or diabetes. Discussing the plan with your doctor, nutritionist, or another health-care professional can be critical.

Certain ailments and medications call for you to eat certain foods for proper nutrition or avoid certain foods so you don't complicate your illness. For example, for someone taking blood-thinning medication, the typical recommendation would be to avoid large doses of vitamin K because it does just the opposite of what these medications intend to do—it actually increases the body's ability to form blood clots. Doctors will rarely tell you to cut out vitamin K altogether, but they will tell you to be aware of how much you're consuming and thus limit your intake of foods such as kale, spinach, collards, broccoli, Swiss chard, Brussels sprouts, and mustard greens. So if the program you're interested in following calls for lots of salads and leafy green vegetables, this would not be the best program for you given that you are taking blood-thinning medications.

You also need to be careful of supplements and how they might interact with food and medications you're taking. Many people don't realize that some supplements are just like taking prescription medications. They can impact your body's biochemistry and physiology, just like a drug you purchase at the pharmacy. Your doctor needs to know what supplements you're taking and whether the program you're considering would be a good fit based on the nutritional suggestions within the plan.

Last, but certainly not least, the safety of a program must be of paramount importance. With thousands of diets on the market and promises of dramatic weight loss requiring extreme measures, it's never a bad idea to have an expert's eyes run over the program to make sure it is nutritionally sound and not potentially health threatening. Marketing has a way of making the most severe, potentially harmful programs seem benign, when in actuality, credible health experts can quickly point out the dangers and risks associated with them. If you have a history of heart disease or inflammatory joint disease like arthritis, maybe the exercise requirement of the program is too much for your body to handle, and you need something less vigorous that can be modified without compromising the results. Seeking out that second opinion, even if it means delaying the start of your weight loss journey, could actually be an important caution that can prevent an injury and get you to your goals faster.

SAFETY

Unless you fall into the very small category of people who will lose weight at any cost, even if it means sacrificing their health, then your number one filter for any program you ultimately select should be its safety. What does it matter that you lose thirty pounds if you're lying in bed throwing up all the time or your kidneys stop working correctly because you've drowned them in so much protein? What does it matter if you can fit into an outfit you haven't worn in two years if it means your hormones are off and your liver is suffering? Choosing the right program is all about understanding and making priorities, and safety should top the list.

In most cases, it's all about using common sense. You don't need a medical degree to sniff out most programs that aren't safe. Any program that has you taking injections, loading up on supplements, only drinking your calories, or allowing you to consume an unlimited amount of fats should raise a red flag. Any program that says you can lose thirty pounds in thirty days or cut your body fat percentage in half in a month should get those alarm bells ringing. If you find yourself going to five different stores to find some must-have ingredient that you've never heard of before or whose name you can't pronounce, it doesn't mean the plan is ineffective or unsafe, but it does mean you need to do your homework and approach it with a fair degree of caution. Before starting any program, especially one that gives you pause, talk to a health expert to get their opinion on whether there are some concerns that you're not seeing or hidden dangers that haven't been well explained.

AFFORDABILITY

What good is a program if you can't afford the food or the exercises require a gym membership or personal trainer that fall out of your budget? Take a long look at the program's requirements and ask yourself whether the expense involved is something you can handle. Carefully read through the plan and do a back-of-the-napkin calculation by estimating all the food, shakes, and smoothies you will need to consume in the week, then estimate what the cost might be.

There are some programs that have a rather rigorous requirement for herbal supplements. These supplements are not only costly, but often they are unnecessary and don't actually deliver the amounts of vitamins and minerals claimed by the manufacturers in their loud advertising. This is not to say that all supplements are expensive or that all of them are shams, but the supplement industry is a multibillion-dollar industry largely unregulated by the Food and Drug Administration. If the program you're considering relies heavily on supplements, then you need to be cautious and a conservative consumer. Read all the fine print, do as much research as you can on your own, and consult with a credible, objective health expert to determine whether they are necessary and worthwhile.

There's no better place to invest your money than in your own health. Making a healthy lifestyle a financial priority is not only prudent but extremely rewarding, as it can help you achieve a longer and better-quality life. But you need to look at the costs and assess whether they are something your resources will allow you to handle. Too many people are excited to start a program, but they do so blindly, only to discover their wallet isn't big enough to handle all of the requirements.

KNOW YOUR DIETING HISTORY

Most people at some point in their lives have been on some type of eating plan to either lose weight (even if it's a small amount), improve a medical condition (like diabetes), increase their energy, or just to improve their overall health. Whatever your experience has been is extremely valuable in moving forward in the right direction. No one knows your body better than you do, and no one knows your ups and downs, hits and misses, better than you either.

Take a few moments and mentally catalog or even write down brief takeaways from programs you've tried in the past. For each program, dedicate one column for things that worked for you while on the plan, then in the next column list those things that didn't work. An honest assessment of these items is critical, as this will better inform what type of program has the best chance of working for you in the future.

Here are some of the questions you need to ask yourself about your previous efforts:

1. Were the food choices okay or were they too restrictive for your liking?
2. Given your schedule, did the plan require too much preparation?
3. Were there things about the plan that caused you to lose motivation?

4. Could you afford the foods?
5. Was it too complicated to follow with too many dos and don'ts?
6. Did you often find yourself hungry?
7. Was the program portable? (Could you follow it away from home?)

Take these answers for the different plans that you tried and create a list of the elements of potential programs that would work for you. While you might not find a plan that perfectly matches, there are enough plans out there that something should certainly come close. Remember, the right diet isn't the one that just promises big results, but the one you can actually do. It should give you a little challenge, but it should be something that you can carry out at no great cost financially or from a time perspective. The right program should not make you unhappy and frustrated and angry at the world. You should enjoy the program and how it makes you feel both physically and emotionally.

MATCH THE DELIVERABLES WITH YOUR GOALS

What good is it if you're trying to lose thirty-five pounds, but the program you're considering specializes more in lowering your blood sugar levels? What good is it if you're trying to lower your cholesterol levels, but the program you're considering suggests generous portions of red meat and high-fat foods like bacon and pork chops? To find the right program, you must read beyond the headlines and hold a magnifying glass to the small print.

Before you choose a plan you discovered in an influencer's Instagram post, you need to first have a clear vision of what, specifically, you're trying to achieve. Knowing your goals and the timeline in which you want to reach those goals can be valuable input in your decision-making process of choosing the best program. Are you trying to lose body fat? Are you trying to lose weight all over your body? Are you trying to drop your blood sugar levels because you've been diagnosed with pre-diabetes or full-blown diabetes? Are you suffering from poor gut health that you want to improve? Ask yourself these types of questions, then formulate very specific answers. Take those answers and match them against the purported claims of the programs you're considering, and this will better inform your choice.

KNOW YOUR EATING STYLE

What do you like to eat and how do you like to eat it? Sounds like something simple to figure out, but these are things that we don't often give much thought to. We just do it. You need to be very aware of the foods you like, those you don't like, and the compromises you might be willing to make to satisfy the requirements of a specific program. If you are someone who rarely eats vegetables or simply can't stand them, would you be able to make a big enough change to follow a program that relies heavily on vegetarian dishes? If you are not a big fan of meat and you enjoy fruits and vegetables, are you willing to change your eating style to follow a program that calls for lots of animal protein and fats, but little or no carbohydrates? You must be honest when answering these questions, even if the person who sits next to you at work followed the plan and lost fifteen pounds in record time.

We all eat differently and enjoy our foods in different ways. Some people don't like eating a big breakfast. Others like to eat their dinner later in the evening. Some have eclectic palates where they might eat sushi one night, then go for Italian the next—steak for dinner one evening, then a Mediterranean vegetarian meal the next. These are flexible eaters— people who like a broad spectrum of cuisines and are happiest when they can sample them at will. Are you this kind of eater? If you are, then you are going to need a plan that is quite liberal in the choices you can make, one that affords you enough flexibility to continue eating in the style you enjoy. If a program suddenly calls for you to eliminate entire food categories or cuisines, this is not a plan that is going to make you happy or one that you're likely to follow for a long period of time, so this would not be a wise choice.

You also need to understand the type of dieter you

are. Some people want a plan that is extremely specific, one that tells them what they need to eat and exact quantities all the way down to the tablespoon. They don't want to have to put much thought into the plan or what they need to do on it. They want it all spelled out so they can just follow directions. I once worked on a popular weight loss show called *Celebrity Fit Club*. I had written what I thought was an amazing diet book that explained everything from the definition of a calorie to how the body digested protein. It was called *The Take Control Diet* and it had the latest research along with nutrition and exercise tips. In my opinion, it was a perfect diet book, full of vital information that would help the reader understand not only what they were eating but why they were eating it. I was proud and confident when I presented it to the celebrities on the show, because it was full of such valuable information that they could use to become better educated and wiser in their decision making. Well, it turned out to be a complete disaster. The celebrities were kind in their rejection, but clearly told me that while it was a smart book and well written and full of important information, there was simply too much extra information that they didn't need. They didn't want to have to figure out what they should eat from guidelines that looked at fat, protein, and carbohydrate content. They didn't want so much control of their choices. They wanted to be told specifically what they could and couldn't eat. One celebrity said, "Just tell me what to eat and when to eat it and I'll do it." Out of this advice was born the subsequent books *The Fat Smash Diet* and *SHRED: The Revolutionary Diet*, which incorporated the principles of making the program information more relatable, relevant, and specific. Those who followed these programs achieved and continue to achieve great success, because while the plans simplify choices and instructions, they also allow users to customize them to better fit their resources, preferences, and goals.

First identify the type of eater you are, the foods that you will and won't eat, and then carefully look at the potential programs. It's unlikely that any program is going to check off all the boxes and give you all the types and quantities of food that you want, but remain open-minded and find the one that comes closest. You know better than anyone how much you're willing to change, so if a program calls for too much, then it's best to keep searching until you find the right fit.

SUSTAINABILITY

Are you looking for fast, short-term results to get the body you want for an imminent vacation or class reunion? Are you trying to fit into a dress or suit for an important event you're attending next month? For many people, quick and fast is what they are looking to achieve, and this is what is most important to them now. Their priority is not what they look like a year or even six months from now. Their vision and focus are tied to immediate results, and thus this urgency should guide the type of program they choose. Many of these programs that promise super-quick results often are either extreme or very rigid. Don't expect a program that allows you to eat almost whatever you want, while not requiring you to exercise, to deliver rapid weight loss. If you are looking for extraordinary results, then you should expect the program to make extraordinary demands on your time and eating choices.

I'm not passing judgment on someone tying their weight loss motivation to an event or social gathering where they want to look their best. There is at least a little bit of vanity in all of us. But buyer beware, as these rapid weight loss programs are often like making a deal with the devil. They will typically put you through an arduous course of extremes, whether it's consuming a ridiculously low number of daily calories or totally removing an entire food group such as carbohydrates. They might require that you exercise an inordinate amount of time or go long periods of time not eating at all. Once you sign up for a program like this, you must also be prepared to accept the consequences of what it's asking you to do.

If you fall into the other large category of those who want substantial weight loss, but also want to make it sustainable, then you are in the market for an entirely different program. You will avoid programs that have you drinking all of your meals or never eating carbs or loading your plate with burgers, bacon, and steak. You might be able to comply with this type of program for a short period of time, but it's virtually impossible to eat this way forever. You will either get bored of eating the same foods all the time, extremely food sick missing those enjoyable foods you had to eliminate, or physically ill from being malnourished. To meet your goals of choosing a program you can stick to over a long period of time, you need to make sure that what the program requires of you is something that you can truly handle not just for a month or two, but for at least a couple of years.

When you talk about programs with long-term sustainability, you're really looking to make a lifestyle change. This doesn't mean that every day, for the rest of your life, you're going to follow a specific plan and only eat the healthiest of foods and exercise five days a week. This means that you are fundamentally changing how you eat, and while there will be plenty of times that you resort to eating things that you've for the most part given up, your new style of eating keeps these items to a minimum. Let's say you're someone who has always eaten a lot of red meat. You make the decision that to improve your health and lose weight, you want to reduce your red meat intake and increase your fish and poultry consumption. This doesn't mean that you won't have a steak or a burger every once in a while; rather, it means that the vast majority of time you're going to order chicken, fish, or salad.

Before investing in any program, make sure you are clear about your true goals. Ask yourself if you're fine with just short-term results that will go away the minute you stop following the plan or if you want to make a wholesale lifestyle change that will deliver long-term results that you will be able to maintain.

NUTRITIONALLY SOUND

While you might not be a nutritionist, it's important to have a basic understanding of whether the nutritional elements of a program make sense. The core of your analysis should be the universally accepted federal guidelines as they pertain to the major nutrients of protein, carbohydrate, and fat—also called the macronutrients, because our bodies require them in large amounts. Our body needs these nutrients in the right quantities, not only to survive, but for peak function. While the body is able to temporarily compensate for short periods of time when we are deficient in a particular nutrient, it shouldn't and can't go for long stretches in this nutritionally deprived state.

So how much of these macronutrients should you be eating on a daily basis? The long-trusted algorithm determines these quantities in relation to the amount of calories you are consuming per day. For example, if you consume 2,000 calories in a day, you should break those calories up into protein, carbohydrate, and fat. Federal guidelines recommend that 10 to 35% of your calories come from protein. That means 200 to 700 calories should come from protein. Fat should contribute 20 to 35% of your calories. That would mean 400 to 700 calories would be linked to fat. (Yes, fat is important, and your body needs it. But you should choose predominantly healthy fats—mono- and polyunsaturated—as well as omega-3 and omega-6 that you can find in foods such as avocados, cheese, fish like salmon, mackerel, and trout, along with nuts that include almonds, walnuts, and macadamia). Carbs are the biggest fuel source for the body. Guidelines recommend that 45 to 65% of your calories come from this important macronutrient, which means 900 to 1,300 calories. (Keep this in mind when you hear about these supposedly great programs that are requiring you to completely eliminate carbs or drastically reduce them!)

These guidelines weren't created by a couple of scientists sitting around an empty lab bench with nothing better to do. Rather lengthy research and analyses have made these numeric recommendations based on their predictive value for disease. As you weigh your options and compare plans when you read the recommendations of the more extreme programs, keep in mind an article published by Harvard Medical School that reported that diets that are less than 45% carbohydrates or more than 35% protein are difficult to follow and tend to be no more effective than other diet programs. Very-low-carbohydrate diets could possibly increase the risk for heart disease, worsen kidney function, and have a negative effect on mood.

It's vital to also consider vitamins, minerals, and other phytonutrients (plant nutrients) that you need. Most people who do not have a chronic illness and eat reasonably well most of the time actually won't need to take multivitamins or supplements. Despite all of the advertising and marketing hype lauding the benefits of supplements, by most estimates, we consume far more than we actually need, since most of what we need we can get right at the table. There are, however, people who might benefit from modest supplementation: the elderly, sufferers of chronic illness, and those who consistently consume a nutritionally depleted diet (fast food with few vegetables four or five times a week as the primary source of nutrition).

Be cautious of programs that forbid basic and plentiful resources such as fruits and vegetables. These are the biggest supply of carbohydrates, the macronutrient that our body really needs in large quantities. Keto-style programs that allow unlimited amounts of red meat and fried fatty foods are another cause for concern, as you will not be consuming enough vitamins and minerals to meet your daily requirements. Keto is not a new concept and has been around for decades, just labeled with different names. Often these programs will suggest you take supplements, clearly because you won't be getting what you need in the food choices or restrictions they're recommending. These programs are also considered to be unsafe over the long term, because they can raise cholesterol levels and, according to some studies, are associated with an increased risk of diabetes. Some studies have even suggested that people on the lowest-carb diets that are high in animal proteins have the highest risk of dying from cancer, cardiovascular conditions, and all other causes. Doctors are also concerned about the impact that extremely high levels of protein can have on kidney function, especially those who might have underlying reduced kidney function and not know it.

Like the old saying goes, "If it sounds too good to be true, it probably is." Many programs will make all kinds of promises, but when you start reading what you need to do to achieve these results, you realize that there are some potentially health-threatening actions you're being asked to take. You can never be too cautious when evaluating a plan on its nutritional merits. What good is losing weight or getting that six-pack when you're damaging your internal organs in the process of reaching that goal?

DIET CHEAT SHEET

DIET TYPE	FLEXIBLE	SUSTAINABLE	NUTRITIONALLY SOUND
High Protein/ High Fat (Keto)	No	No	No
Low Fat	Yes	Maybe	Yes
Low Carb	No	Maybe	Yes
Raw	Maybe	No	Yes
Vegetarian	Maybe	Yes	Yes
Intermittent Fasting	Maybe	Yes	Yes
Clean Eating	Yes	Yes	Yes

Glossy advertisements and eye-popping internet headlines are not how anyone should choose a diet program. Because we all gain and lose weight differently and have unique tastes in foods, successful plans for others might not be the right fit. Remember that very well constructed plans can still be ineffective if they're not the right match for you. Too many people in either desperation or excitement select a program without giving it the necessary amount of thought it takes to make a sound decision. Be honest about what you're looking to achieve and the kind of plan that will push you but is still doable. When you're patient and thoughtful you'll give yourself the best shot at winning.

⇉ ACTION PLAN ⇇

1. Select 3 eating different plans. Describe the basic elements of each. Talk to a health expert about their safety and feasibility. _____

_____

_____

_____

_____

_____

_____

_____

_____

2. Make a short list of things that have worked for you on previous eating plans and what didn't. _____

_____

_____

_____

_____

_____

_____

_____

_____

3. Write down a realistic time that it will take for you to reach your goals, then see which plan gives you the best chance at achieving them. _____

_____

4. Decide what style of eater and dieter you are: flexible or rigid? _____

_____

5. Decide if you're looking for short-term or long-term results or both. _____

_____

6. Use the diet cheat sheet to determine the category of diet that best fits you. _____

_____

7. Create a quick weekly budget of how much you're willing to spend on food and exercise. _____

_____

_____

_____

_____

_____

_____

_____

4

CRUSH THE CRAVINGS

Listen to your body. Most of the time it already has the answers.

Almost everyone at some point experiences a food or drink craving, whether it's a hankering for a big piece of rich chocolate cake or a slice of pizza with ice-cold soda. For many, these cravings occur daily and provide yet another complication in an already complicated journey to lose weight and keep it off. Unfortunately, the frequency and depth of these cravings can prove to be insurmountable for many and result in "cheating" or going off a plan they've been committed to following. In a nutshell, these cravings can be an absolute dietary disaster and a major contributor to weight loss failure.

Let's take a step back and look at what food cravings are and how they develop. Food cravings are defined as an intense desire to eat a specific foodstuff. People often confuse hunger and cravings. There is an important distinction to be made. Hunger is a sensation we get when our body tells us that it needs nourishment to meet its energetic needs. Hunger itself is not specific; rather, the body is just saying, "I need food." But a craving is very specific and very intentional. According to Kent Berridge, a professor of psychology and neuroscience at the University of Michigan, "Hunger is an input to the brain's craving system; it can amplify the craving system." He goes on to say that the hunger system and craving system have some differences and can work slightly separate from each other.

Scientists have been able to figure out that cravings have physical, physiologic, and psychological underpinnings. It was believed for a long time that people craved foods based on what the body needed. That logic went something like this: your body is deficient in vitamin A, so you develop a craving for carrots or sweet potatoes, which are both high in vitamin A. Further research has shown that while in some cases there might be a relationship between what you crave and what your body nutritionally needs, the vast majority of cravings have no basis whatsoever in your body's nutritional deficiencies. The answer really lies in the brain.

When we eat food that tastes good and makes us feel good, a system of chemical messaging occurs in the brain that increases the likelihood we will seek this food out in the future and derive more pleasure. This is all based on the brain's reward system, which also happens to be at the center of cravings. There are several areas in the center of the brain (including the nucleus accumbens, ventral tegmental area, and prefrontal cortex) that are important to eliciting pleasure and driving us to seek more of that pleasure. When you eat food that you like, your brain releases a chemical called dopamine. Dopamine is classified as a neurotransmitter, because it is a chemical messenger created and released in our brains that exchanges communication among nerve cells.

It's like nerve language—the nerve cells are like our mouth, and dopamine is like the words that come out of our mouth. Once you eat a food that you like, certain areas of the brain release dopamine. This dopamine travels to other areas of the brain that do several things: (1) tell you that the experience was pleasurable, (2) activate the brain's memory centers so that they pay close attention to all features of that rewarding experience so that it can be repeated at a future time, and (3) help you establish an association between environmental cues and whether or not that experience was rewarding.

Let's say you like fried dough or funnel cake with lots of powdered sugar sprinkled on it. Maybe your first experience eating that delicious fried dough was at a local fair. Once you bite into it and enjoy the taste, the dopamine goes wild in your brain, telling you how great it was and recording all the sights, smells, and sounds that were associated with that pleasurable experience. The next time you are at a fair or similar atmosphere like a carnival, even with your stomach already full, you develop this desire to get a piece of that sugary fried dough. You're not hungry, but you suddenly have a craving for it.

This reward system and its various mechanisms that influence cravings are very similar to what is found with substance addiction, particularly drugs like heroin and cocaine. Scientists have looked at brain imaging studies and found that cravings and drug addiction light up similar regions in the brain that are involved in learning, memory, and motivation. The good news, however, about food cravings is that eventually, if you don't give into them, they will pass. (This is not the same for hunger. More on this later.) So the key for anyone who is embarking on a weight loss plan and has to restrict or eliminate some of the "fun" foods they're accustomed to eating, is to be able to survive the craving or avoid the environmental stimuli that produce them.

First, discover what stimuli are associated with your cravings. For example, when you get upset at your boss, you might try to relieve that stress by going to the vending machine and buying a bag of barbecue potato chips. Experience has taught you that not only do the chips taste great but they take your mind off the anger you're feeling toward your boss. Driving a certain route home that takes you past your favorite fast-food restaurant will expose you to the stimulus for your craving. Whether it's seeing the sign or the long line of cars waiting at the drive-thru window or the savory smells floating through your open window, you are likely to encounter a cue that kicks that reward-seeking loop into high gear. If you know you're vulnerable to these cues, taking that route to drive home is not the best idea.

There have been thousands of studies addressing food cravings, their basis, how they're connected to the body's chemistry, and how they can best be handled. Two salient findings of these studies are worth noting, as they can be informative in how you choose to handle your cravings. First, after looking at the various types of foods that people crave, researchers found that the most commonly craved were salty snacks or sweets high in sugar and fat. But regardless of which type of food was craved, the common characteristic about the foods was that they all tended to be high in calories. People don't typically crave raw carrots or celery sticks.

The second finding worth noting is the influence of the type of diet that's consumed and the likelihood that you will experience cravings. Researchers found that people who consumed a more monotonous diet—consistently eating most of the same foods with little diversity—tended to report significantly more cravings than those who ate a variety of foods. The body tends to miss what it's accustomed to consuming but suddenly is not getting. This is instructive as you decide which diet plan you choose to follow. Be cautioned that choosing one with numerous food restrictions could mean you'll be battling more cravings, which can make an already challenging journey even more difficult.

Research has also shown that cravings have an expiration, whereas hunger does not. Hunger is controlled by the body's physiologic need to be nourished with energy in the form of calories and other nutrients that are critical for survival and functioning. Think of your body as a car. When you are low on fuel or oil, a light flashes on your dashboard to let you know that you are close to empty and it's important to refuel or add more oil. This light stays on until you've taken the appropriate actions to address the problem. There's no button you can push to make it go away, and it won't turn off by itself if you simply wait it out. If you turn off the car and park it for a week, once you turn it back on, the light is still going to come on and stay on, because this is a critical problem that needs to be addressed as soon as possible. Your hunger is your body's light coming on telling you that it needs nourishment.

Imagine another scenario where you get into your car and your cell phone's Bluetooth feature is turned on. The car recognizes your device and wording flashes on your front display asking if you want to connect your phone to the car's Bluetooth system. If you want to connect, you press a button and the car and phone are connected. If you don't see the message or simply don't push the button, after a couple of minutes, the prompt will go away on its own. The Bluetooth prompt from your car is the same as your food craving. If you don't respond to the craving, after a period of time, unlike hunger, it will go away.

Keeping yourself active and distracted when a craving comes is a very effective technique for preventing yourself from giving in to the urge. Whether you choose to do something physical like go for a walk or do some jumping jacks or engage your mind by listening to music or an interesting podcast, cravings can be managed and, in many instances, bypassed. The answer starts in your belief system. You must believe that regardless of how deep and forceful the craving, you can get beyond it and be better off by not giving in to it. Following are nine things you can do right away to outlast your cravings:

EAT MINDFULLY

The process of mindful eating is all about helping you gain control over your eating habits. Studies have shown that this technique can help with weight loss, sticking to a plan, and reducing binge eating. The idea is that you want to reach a state of full attention to your eating experience. Try this simple exercise for mindful eating. Once your food is served or plated, let it sit there for a moment before digging in. Look at all of the food and the colors. Smell the aromas and see if you can distinguish which foods and ingredients are producing them. Next, give some thought to what you're eating and why you're eating it and what it could be doing to your body or diet journey. Be present while you eat by slowing down, chewing thoroughly, and really trying to taste all the flavors and feel all the textures of the individual ingredients and spices. Being mindful can help you distinguish between hunger and a craving, and this can help you choose a better response rather than impulsively grabbing for food just because you crave it.

⇒ MINDFUL EATING TECHNIQUES ⇐

+ Appreciate your food.
+ Pay attention to the effects particular foods have on your feelings and body.
+ Engage as many of your senses as possible by noticing colors, sounds, textures, smells, and tastes.
+ Eat with the intention of maintaining or improving your overall health.

STAY HYDRATED

It's not uncommon for thirst to be confused with hunger or food cravings. You don't have to run five miles and stand dripping in sweat for your body to be thirsty and in need of water. We lose water throughout the day in ways other than sweating. These imperceptible water losses make us thirsty, but we might perceive this thirst as hunger or a craving for a specific food. Water is extremely important, because it does everything from improving digestion and elimination to fueling our cells and helping us feel energized. Studies have shown that drinking enough water before a meal can help you feel full faster, which can reduce appetite and help with weight loss. The next time you have a craving, try drinking 8 to 12 ounces of water and see if the craving diminishes or goes away.

CONTROL YOUR ENVIRONMENT

If you don't have it, you can't eat it. Controlling your food environment and eliminating temptation or cues that will trigger a craving is essential. Make it as difficult for yourself as possible to access the forbidden foods and drinks. Don't bring into your house those items that you are not supposed to eat. The people you live with might like and want something that you are not supposed to eat, so you have to make a decision. If you know that the food sitting in the cabinet or refrigerator is only going to spark a craving, then have a conversation with your housemates about how important it is for you not to be around that particular food or drink and ask that they help out by agreeing that it's alright not to have it in the house. When you're at work, stay away from the trouble spots in the cafeteria or avoid walking by the vending machines. You won't always be able to control your environment, but whenever you can, do your best.

Eat Protein

One of the causes for cravings is an imbalance of blood sugar levels. When blood sugars rise quickly, then fall, this makes you vulnerable to cravings. Researchers used brain imaging scans and found that small drops in the level of blood sugar activated a region of the brain that produces a desire to eat. However, when the blood sugar levels were adequate, the region of the brain that controls impulses was activated. This is about the tug of war that happens in our subconscious between our ability to control our cravings and our inability to resist foods we really shouldn't be eating. Maintaining consistent blood sugar levels can help you win this battle, and protein can be part of the solution.

Protein is important to our body for many reasons, including building muscle, producing hormones, and nourishing the nervous system, among many other functions. However, its role in balancing blood sugar levels is critical to holding off cravings. It takes the body more time to digest protein than carbohydrates. In fact, most protein-rich foods have a much lower glycemic index than carbohydrates, which means they cause a much slower rise of blood sugar levels, something that is important in reducing cravings.

REDUCE STRESS

Research has shown that stress may actually prompt food cravings and be influential in determining eating behaviors. People tend to experience more cravings and eat more calories when they are stressed. Stress also has a true physical effect on the body, particularly when it comes to cortisol, the body's main stress hormone. Cortisol is made and released by the small adrenal glands located at the top of your kidneys. When your body is stressed, the adrenal glands release it to counteract that stress. Cortisol does this by doing several things, including regulating blood pressure, increasing blood sugar levels, boosting energy levels, and managing how the body uses carbohydrates, proteins, and fats. Excessive cortisol can cause you to gain weight, especially in the belly.

Cortisol is connected to your body's desire to seek out rewards, and sometimes these rewards come in the form of comfort foods that typically are not permitted on most weight loss plans. You could be having a really bad day at work that leads to you feeling stressed out and under pressure. Your body responds by releasing cortisol into your bloodstream. Foods that are full of sugar and fat put an abrupt halt to this escalating cycle of stress because they light up the pleasure center in your brain and make you feel happy. This happiness overcomes the anxiety and stress you were feeling, and your brain now has created an important pathway or stress-escape route that can be easily found and used again if needed. The food you've eaten—whether it's a piece of cake or french fries—now gets recorded as a solution to your stress.

Sometimes the key to overcoming your cravings is identifying your stressor early and addressing it before you start craving that piece of pie or chocolate fudge. Everyone has their own stress relievers, but here are some you might try.

1. Listen to music you enjoy.
2. Exercise or go for a short walk.
3. Watch a video of something you find entertaining.
4. Call a friend or loved one and have a pleasant conversation.

5. Light a candle with calming scents such as lavender, orange blossom, geranium, rose, or bergamot.
6. Find a quiet place where you can close your eyes and meditate.
7. Play with your pet.

There are many types of meditation exercises you can employ to reduce stress, but one simple one is sitting in a position of comfort with your back straight, feet flat on the floor or your legs crossed, and eyes closed. Rest your hands in your lap. As you slowly breathe through your nose, clear your mind of any thoughts and focus on the process of your breath moving in and out of your body. Try to visualize the molecules of air and their movement into your nose, down the back of your throat and into your lungs. If your meditative state of connectedness is interrupted by physical sensations or thoughts, make sure you make note of this, then bring your focus back to the process and experience of breathing.

GET SOME SLEEP

We are just at the tip of the iceberg in really understanding how sleep (or lack of it) influences our internal physiology. What scientists do know, however,
is that sleep deprivation can actually disrupt our hormonal balances and lead to fluctuations that cause
poor appetite control and strong cravings. Studies
have shown that when participants did not get enough
sleep and were flashed pictures of health-conscious
food versus junk food, the pictures of the junk food
activated the reward centers in their brains. The more
tired we are, the more likely we are to make unhealthy
food choices, when what we really need is more sleep.

A University of Chicago study looked at sleep
deprivation and its relationship to food choices. The
researchers found that the otherwise healthy participants who were deprived of an appropriate amount
of sleep were unable to resist what researchers called
"highly palatable, rewarding snacks," which were classified as cookies, candy, and chips, despite the fact that
just two hours prior, they had eaten a meal that con-
tained 90% of their daily caloric needs. Researchers

discovered that sleep restriction boosted a chemical called endocannabinoid 2-arachidonoylglcerol (2-AG) that was typically at low levels during the night and early morning. When the level of this chemical rose, the study participants reported higher scores for hunger and a stronger desire to eat. They were given the opportunity to consume snacks and they tended to eat nearly twice as much fat compared to when they had snacks after sleeping a full eight hours.

Many people think they are getting enough sleep when they are not. Getting up in the middle of the night, constantly changing the number of sleep hours you get each night, or not getting sound sleep can contribute to this undesirable state of sleep deprivation. Improve your sleep habits and there's a strong chance you will improve your ability to resist foods that your body doesn't need but feels like it must have.

POUR SOME TEA

Sometimes simply outlasting the craving can be an effective strategy to not give in to your urges. When you get a craving, go through the simple, calming, step-by-step process of brewing your own tea. By the time you've gone through all the steps and are ready to drink the tea, there's a good chance the craving will have subsided. There are certain spices you can add to your tea that can be effective at helping you balance your blood sugar levels. Cinnamon, ginger, and turmeric might help do the trick.

DON'T SKIP MEALS

Hunger feeds our cravings, so it's important that you don't allow yourself to go for long periods of time without eating. Skipping meals is a big culprit when it comes to developing cravings, because rather than just being slightly hungry (as is the case when you might skip just a snack), you are now ravenous. This deep hunger is a danger for those trying to stick to a weight loss plan. First, you are more likely to develop cravings. Second, you are vulnerable to grabbing and eating anything that will help satisfy the hunger. Smart snacking on foods rich in protein and fiber (not sugary snacks) will help you keep your blood sugar levels stable and prevent intense hunger from developing.

FILL UP ON CHROMIUM

Chromium is an essential trace element that once ingested can enhance the effect of insulin and help lower blood glucose levels, causing them to remain stable. There is no universally recommended dietary allowance for this element, but some researchers suggest 1,000 micrograms a day should be the upper limit. While chromium is available in supplements, you can get all you need naturally from foods. Vegetables such as green beans, broccoli, and potatoes are rich in chromium. Other good sources include beef and poultry, milk and dairy products, whole grains like oats, and fruits like apples and bananas.

The table below is a quick cheat sheet of suggestions for how to address your craving with foods that will also give you more nutritional benefit with fewer calories. Try to keep some of these readily available so that you are prepared when the craving strikes.

CRAVING	SUBSTITUTION
SUGAR/SWEET	Fruit (mangoes, pineapple, grapes, berries)
	Dark chocolate (contains more than 70% cocoa)
	Sugar-free chewing gum or mints
	Sweet potatoes
	Raw broccoli and hummus
	Dates
	Raw carrots
	Frozen chocolate bananas
	All-fruit ice pop (puree your favorite fruit with lime juice, put a stick in it, and freeze)
	Baked apple (stuffed with nuts or oats)
	Hot chocolate (limit the amount of chocolate syrup)

cont.

CRAVING	SUBSTITUTION
SALTY	Sea salt crackers and nut butter
	Diced watermelon with crumbled feta cheese and balsamic vinegar
	Low-fat mozzarella cheese sticks and olives
	Dill pickles
	Edamame with a light sprinkle of sea salt
	Tomatoes with crumbled feta cheese and olive oil
	Sesame seaweed snacks
	Turkey jerky

Everyone has cravings. Don't feel guilty or abnormal because a food pops into your mind at the strangest of times. Cravings don't always follow a predictable schedule. Getting your cravings under control, however, can be an important tipping point in your struggle to eat better, lose weight, and keep it off. You must know yourself to decide what the best route will be to handle your cravings, as we all process them differently and have different coping skills that can keep them in check. If a craving is too difficult and too distracting to ignore, confront it with an effective strategy that will either crush it or keep it at bay.

⇉ ACTION PLAN ⇇

1. List your most common cravings. _____
_____
_____
_____
_____
_____
_____

2. List the most common circumstances and/or times
you seem to get your cravings. _____
_____
_____
_____
_____
_____
_____

3. Decide on 3 strategies you will try at first to crush your
cravings. _____
_____
_____
_____
_____

_____

_____

_____

4. Keep the unhealthy foods you crave out of your house and out of reach.

5. Spend an entire week eating every meal mindfully.

6. For an entire week, keep a craving journal. Make sure you record the food craved, the time, the circumstances surrounding the craving, and how long it lasted. _____

_____

_____

_____

_____

_____

7. Stock your kitchen and workplace with cravings swaps.

5

BOOST YOUR CONFIDENCE

*Motivation will get you to start,
confidence will get you to finish.*

The process of embarking and progressing on a weight loss journey is a microcosm of life itself. There is trepidation mixed with uncertainty, setbacks giving birth to intense moments of doubt, and struggle leading to victory. Successful weight loss requires you to be fully equipped and prepared to deal with not only what has been predicted, but the unforeseen as well, for it is typically what you're not expecting that can prove to be your biggest obstacle. One of the most powerful weapons in your weight loss arsenal is your confidence, and how you employ it can be the deciding factor in whether you succeed or not.

Confidence is the belief in one's self and one's ability to succeed. Confidence and motivation work in tandem. The more confident you are in your ability to succeed, the more motivated you will be to stick to your plan and ultimately reach your goals. We all have different levels of self-confidence, and there are different things in our life experiences that either build it up or tear it down. But possessing confidence is critical, as studies have shown that people with a healthy level of confidence have happier relationships, earn more money, and are generally more successful at reaching the goals they set for themselves. People who are more confident tend to be more competent, and others around them not only can sense this, but can help clear a path to success that once seemed clogged and too difficult to navigate.

Often, self-confidence is mistakenly confused with self-esteem. Self-confidence is focused more on how you feel about your ability to do or accomplish a task, whereas self-esteem is your overall feeling about yourself. A well-known illustration of high self-esteem is the image of a kitten looking in the mirror, and the image appearing in the mirror is that of an adult lion. While self-esteem and self-confidence have their distinctions, they are intimately linked, and in many instances collaborate to influence our ability to perform certain tasks. People with high self-esteem tend to have higher levels of confidence and find more success in the things they do. The noted self-improvement guru Dr. Max Maltz once said, "Low self-esteem is like driving through life with your hand brake on." The good news is that you can improve your self-esteem, and this inherently translates into a boost of confidence. But first, there are questions you need to answer to get a better sense of your confidence and your ability to follow your program well enough to get the results you seek:

1. Have you ever failed at a diet plan in the past, and if so, what do you think caused the failure?
2. Do you feel confident that you can lose weight and keep the weight off?

3. How does your weight affect your feelings of self-worth?

4. Do you feel like you have the discipline to do what it takes to stick to the plan?

5. Are your goals realistic, and do you think you'll be able to reach them?

Answering those introductory questions is all about helping you explore your true thoughts and innermost feelings. This process of establishing self-awareness is critical, because it helps you identify potential issues that might hinder your journey as well as things that can facilitate success. It's also critical that you're aware of your self-esteem, because trying to boost your confidence might also mean boosting your self-esteem. First, let's take stock of your self-esteem, as feeling good about who you are and what you are is the seed from which all else grows. There are several methods to assess self-esteem, but one that is popular and easy to perform is the Rosenberg self-esteem scale that was developed by sociologist Morris Rosenberg in 1965 and all these years later is still widely used. Answer the questions and see where you fall on the self-esteem scale.

Rosenberg Self-Esteem Scale Instructions

1. Answer the following 10 items on a 4-point scale that ranges from Strongly Agree to Strongly Disagree.

2. To score your answers, assign a value to each of the 10 items accordingly:

   For items 1, 2, 4, 6, 7: Strongly Agree=3, Agree=2, Disagree=1, Strongly Disagree=0

   For items 3, 5, 8, 9, 10: Strongly Agree=0, Agree=1, Disagree=2, Strongly Disagree=3

3. The scoring scale ranges from 0 to 30, with 30 being the highest possible score. Scores that fall below 15 indicate low self-esteem. The higher your score, the higher your self-esteem.

Below you will find a list of statements that deal with your general feelings about yourself. If you strongly agree, circle SA. If you agree with the statement, circle A. If you disagree, circle D. If you strongly disagree circle SD.

	STRONGLY AGREE	AGREE	DISAGREE	STRONGLY DISAGREE
1. I feel that I'm a person of worth, at least on an equal plane with others.	SA	A	D	SD
2. I feel that I have a number of good qualities.	SA	A	D	SD
3. All in all, I'm inclined to feel that I'm a failure.	SA	A	D	SD
4. I am able to do things as well as most other people.	SA	A	D	SD
5. I feel I do not have much to be proud of.	SA	A	D	SD

Mind over Weight

	STRONGLY AGREE	AGREE	DISAGREE	STRONGLY DISAGREE
6. I take a positive attitude toward myself.	SA	A	D	SD
7. On the whole, I am satisfied with myself.	SA	A	D	SD
8. I wish I could have more respect for myself.	SA	A	D	SD
9. I certainly feel useless at times.	SA	A	D	SD
10. At times I think I am no good at all.	SA	A	D	SD

SELF-EFFICACY

In the field of behavioral psychology, there's a well-studied concept called self-efficacy. This term is used to describe the way we believe in our ability to meet challenges that lie ahead of us and reach our goals. Someone who feels confident that they will be able to reach their goals has high self-efficacy. Someone who is uncertain and lacks confidence in their ability to carry out a specific task and reach a specific goal has a low self-efficacy. Why does this matter? Research has consistently found a strong link between self-efficacy and success. As it pertains to dieting, studies have suggested that one's self-efficacy is a great predictor of dieting success or failure. If you have doubts from the outset about the likelihood of your success in losing weight and reaching your goals, then it's like jumping into a pool with one hand tied behind your back. If you have great skill and endurance, and some luck, you can survive, but the odds are heavily stacked in favor of your not faring so well if one hand remains tied behind your back. People who approach diets from a position of high self-efficacy are more likely not to succumb to the obstacles they face and are more likely to find ways to adjust and do what's necessary to ultimately reach their goals.

Interestingly, your self-efficacy (self-belief) is related to your self-esteem (self-worth). A high self-efficacy can boost your self-esteem, and a high self-esteem can increase your confidence in your ability to carry out tasks and reach goals. There is, however, one important distinction. The concept of self-esteem centers on a person's "being," while the concept of self-efficacy focuses on the state of "doing."

Many people have the skill set, knowledge, or a sufficient enough plan to accomplish what they set out to do; however, it's often their lack of confidence that's holding them back from succeeding. Unfortunately, many don't even recognize that they suffer from low confidence. If you don't know something is broken, then you won't know it needs to be fixed. Read carefully through this list of signs that you might lack confidence. Awareness is always the first step in the process of change.

⇜ SIGNS YOU LACK CONFIDENCE ⇝

+ Feeling compelled to always explain yourself or your decisions
+ Constantly complaining and blaming others for something that is wrong
+ Difficulty accepting compliments from others; you downplay what they say or flat-out deny it
+ Constantly searching for/needing approval from others for validation
+ Socially withdrawn, often avoiding others or making excuses to get out of social events
+ Overly defensive
+ Low expectations of what you can and will accomplish
+ Feeling embarrassed or shame when you don't achieve perfection
+ Unable to enjoy the present, because you fear the future
+ You consistently back down during disagreements, even when you feel strongly about something

+ The possibility of change causes you some level of anxiety and stress
+ You often exhibit defensive body language such as folding your arms
+ Magnify criticism directed at you and respond immediately and aggressively
+ Constantly offering apologies, often for things that don't even necessitate one
+ Feel the need to constantly inject self-deprecating humor into the conversation or an awkward situation

BUILD YOUR CONFIDENCE

You've certainly heard the expression that someone is "naturally confident." Well, legions of scientists have looked at this concept and, as with many scientific principles, can't seem to agree on whether it is accurate. Some believe that some of us are born with genes that predispose us to develop great self-confidence, while others believe that self-confidence is not something prewired in your DNA, but something that can be learned and constructed as we grow and evolve in the world. Regardless of which school of thought you subscribe to, everyone agrees that confidence can be boosted. It's important to remember, however, that while having a high confidence level can be extremely helpful when starting a program and trying to stick to it, too much confidence can actually work against you. Overconfidence can breed arrogance that not only puts you in the wrong mind-set for the tasks ahead but can cloud your vision and willingness to do what is required to succeed. In this chapter, we will focus on eleven simple strategies that you can use to boost your confidence and improve your self-efficacy, making you better equipped to tackle the challenges of weight loss and succeed.

1. **VISUALIZE WHO YOU WANT TO BE.** Visualization employs our imagination to use mental imagery to create visions of the things we want and how to make them happen. Golfers often talk about closing their eyes right before swinging the club and visualizing the desired flight of the golf ball. Actors

talk about how they visualize their scenes before participating in them, seeing themselves onstage and hearing themselves deliver their lines. Some people will take time to visualize what they will look like after weight loss or the home they will build after they secure a lucrative job. There is a large body of evidence that has linked the power of visualization to successful attainment of one's goals. In fact, some researchers found that the more detailed your vision of success, the more confident you will feel about attaining it. Imagine yourself wearing a particular outfit or standing in the mirror after a shower and the improvements you will be able to see. Let your mind see the change first, then let your actions deliver results.

2. **SILENCE THE OPINIONS OF OTHERS.** One of the biggest blows to confidence is relying on external validators. When you allow the opinions of others to influence your sense of self-worth or ability, then you are heading down a tricky road that could ultimately lead to disappointment. Your voice is the most important voice you need to hear, and it needs to be positive and strong. What you think

about yourself and abilities is paramount. It's completely fine when others who have your best interest at heart give you constructive criticism, but you need to make sure that what they're saying or the volume at which they're saying it doesn't erode your confidence. You also need to be mindful that many people who you think might have your best interest at heart might selfishly have only their own interest in mind. It's very important to separate those who are well-meaning and helpful from those who are standing on top of you so that they can appear taller.

Develop a positive inner voice that blocks out the negative chatter you hear from others. Frequently remind yourself of your talents and insist that you will accomplish your goals regardless of how difficult they may be or how long it will take. Even pick a couple of affirmations to repeat: they can be extremely powerful tools to boost your confidence and believe in yourself. Say something like "I have the strength and determination to succeed, and I will not let anyone or anything get in my way" and say it out loud to yourself every day. Remember that the brain only has room for one thought at a time. If that space is occupied with something positive, then there's no room for the negative. When those doubts begin to creep in, simply push them away by thinking optimistically and feeling confident about who you are and what you can accomplish.

3. **HAVE REALISTIC EXPECTATIONS.** You can't build confidence if you constantly feel like you're underachieving. It's important that you attain some level of success early in the process, as this quickly boosts your confidence to go after even loftier goals. If you set unrealistic expectations that are too difficult to achieve, then you're going to find yourself constantly disappointed. Regardless of how enthusiastic you are about succeeding or how optimistic you are that you'll reach your goals, if your expectations are unrealistic, then it's highly unlikely you will be successful. Success begets more success, so start with small, attainable goals and milestones such as losing two pounds in a week or having only three snacks during the course of the day instead of four. You want to make sure that you set yourself up so that you will feel the adrenaline rush of achieving and create momentum that will push you to even more success.

4. **ACKNOWLEDGE YOUR SUCCESS.** Too often we don't recognize or acknowledge our own successes. This doesn't mean you should walk around with a gold star stuck to your forehead, but it does mean you should feel you *deserve* to have one stuck there. We have been conditioned to spend a lot of time focusing on things we need to do and not enough time on things that we've done. It's good to have others recognize your accomplishments, but it's even more important that you do so and take stock of what you've been able to do. Small victories are just as important as large ones, so be willing to acknowledge even the minor accomplishments. Once they've reached their achievements, successful people don't permanently stop and spend the rest of their lives basking in the glory. But they do take the time to temporarily hit the pause button and appreciate what they've been able to accomplish. This inspires them to achieve even more.

5. **ATTACK YOUR FEARS.** Rather than avoid your fears, go ahead and attack them. Even if you don't conquer a fear right away, just the process of

stepping up and confronting what has made you nervous or anxious can help you build confidence. This doesn't mean you should suddenly sign up to go jump out of a plane to attack your fear of heights. It's more effective to start with smaller things first and work your way up. Overcoming fears or being able to lessen their psychological burdens requires a process that you must be willing to trust. This is about your learning and then affirming that the consequences you've always associated with a particular action or situation are not in line with what really will happen. It can take some time for you to get comfortable with this new knowledge and lose your anxiety, so be patient. You might not feel a big difference right away, but be persistent and make sure you're present in the moment and aware of all that you do and feel.

6. **FIND RELIABLE SUPPORT.** When others know what you are trying to do and the challenges these activities or goals might present, they can be a great source of encouragement and support. They can provide a calmer, more objective voice than the one that's shouting in your head that you are not doing well

or that you won't succeed. Make an agreement with your friends and actually write it down. Give them the license to be honest with you when things are good *and* when things are bad. This relationship is based on trust, and you must be willing to listen to what they say and not question them or yourself when they compliment you or see your abilities differently from you. There is an enormous amount of research that shows the benefits of a strong support system, whether you're battling a medical condition or experiencing anguish from a bad relationship. Seeking and establishing a support network is not a sign of weakness, but a sign of strength. If you don't have friends or close family members to turn to, you could join an online support group or fellowship with members of your church or an affinity group comprised of others of similar interests or concerns.

7. **FOCUS ON STRENGTHS.** It's so easy to fall into the trap of focusing your attention on all the things that you don't do well or things going wrong in your life. You don't cook too well or you're a little socially awkward in front of strangers or you're not the most physically coordinated. Beating yourself up

time and again over these perceived shortcomings will serve only to keep your head pushed underneath the waters of negativity. Instead, spend most of your time thinking about your strengths. All of us have strengths. Think about your positive attributes and assets and how you can enhance and broaden them. If you've spent more time in the critique mode, you will be shocked to find out how much there is to cheer about when you switch into the positive-assessment mode. It's important to remind yourself that you have talents just like anyone else. And while they may not be recognized and supported as well as they should be, that doesn't mean they don't exist.

8. **BE KIND TO YOURSELF.** Life is too short to be so hard on yourself. It's okay to have high standards and great expectations, but when making a self-assessment of who you are or what you've done, be kind. We all have a friend or know of someone who spends an inordinate amount of time being self-deprecating or apologizing for things that need no apologies. They constantly slip in bad comments about themselves, whether it's about how they look or how uninteresting

they are. They typically say these things as an aside to a larger conversation, and they say it in a playful way to poke fun at themselves. The reality, however, is that there can be darkness buried underneath this "aw-shucks" façade that gives rise to self-doubt and at times even self-loathing. It's okay to challenge yourself and be constructively critical when you fall short of the mark, but you still need to do it in a way that doesn't do damage. A good model to follow is the relationship you have with a friend who you love and enjoy being around and are relaxed and natural with. Treat yourself like you would treat that friend. There are things you would never say or do to them that you nevertheless feel it's acceptable to do to yourself.

9. **LEVEL THE PLAYING FIELD.** All of us have something we're really good at. Whether it's gardening, sports, trivia, or cooking, we have an above-average skill set that makes us unique in our own way. The mistake that people with low confidence make is overlooking their own value and capabilities and, instead, only emphasizing and applauding what they find in others. A big part of boosting your confi-

dence is having a realistic conversation with yourself about your equality with others. One of your friends may have gotten a PhD in neuroscience and another might be a vice president at a bank. That's wonderful and laudable. But you could be a whiz data analyst or excellent caretaker or exemplary volunteer at a local food pantry. Your friends are not above you; rather you are equals, and it's important that you see it that way. It's completely fine to admire the successes of others and compliment them accordingly, but it's not alright when you do so and feel unequal to the person you're complimenting. When others give you compliments or want to highlight something you've done, don't shy away from that or tell them that it was "no big deal." You have to give yourself permission to feel good about what you do and not be embarrassed when others seek to acknowledge it.

10. **SET BOUNDARIES.** For people who are naturally shy or simply don't like confrontation, it can be difficult to set boundaries with others. Being direct and potentially hurting someone else's feelings can be

uncomfortable. However, you must set boundaries and be more assertive or people will simply do and say what they want whenever the mood strikes them. Saying no can be difficult, but it resonates extremely powerfully with them and within you. It can be an empowering experience if you allow it to be. You can't let others define who and what you are, because not only does that give them power over you but it undercuts your confidence. Standing up for yourself is not rude or aggressive at all. You can do this politely, but with the necessary firmness to let others know that they don't have free rein to do as they please in domains that should be under your control. "I appreciate your concern, but this is a decision I need to make for myself." When you take back what is yours and others learn to respect that, your confidence will rise accordingly. In essence, you are creating neural pathways that automate a response to habitual behaviors. Many people who are overweight because they overeat or can't stop snacking on high-calorie foods, tend to have neural pathways that initiate this behavior that leads to unwanted consequences. The good news is that by changing your thoughts around the stimulating event or situation and then changing your response, you can create new neural pathways which your brain will now use instead of the old ones which eventually are lost.

11. **CREATE OR FIND A MANTRA THAT IN-STILLS CONFIDENCE.** The purpose of practicing something repeatedly is to improve one's ability to perform a task. Whether it's learning a new instrument, improving your tennis serve, or speaking a foreign language, it's the repetition of doing something correctly that not only improves performance, but also increases our confidence that we can carry out the task successfully in the future. The same can be said when it comes to what we hear or think about our abilities. The more we hear or think that we can succeed at something, the more we start believing it, and the more confident we become. Create your own mantras or use some of those below. Write them down and keep them in a place that's easily accessible like your refrigerator or posted on the side of your computer monitor. The more you say it, the more you're likely to believe it.

⇴ CONFIDENCE MANTRAS ⇷

+ No one is perfect. I can make mistakes like anyone and it doesn't make me any less of a person or any less skilled.

+ Failure is a great opportunity for me to learn how to be successful.

+ Each small step I take is a step in the direction of my goals.

+ I will not let others or situations dissuade me from the pursuit of my goals.

+ I am talented regardless of what others think or say.

+ I will not stop until I win.

+ Every day I will do something that makes me better and puts me closer to my goal.

+ No matter how bad a day, the clock runs out at 24 hours.

+ I deserve to be happy.

+ This is my life and I will dream as big as I want.

+ Success is earned, not given.

Confidence will guide and protect you. It will make you strong when you need strength and resilience to bounce back. Confidence is yours, and others don't have a right to diminish or steal it. Hold on to it with great vigor and with no regrets. Never be ashamed to believe in yourself and your vast potential to achieve.

⇥ ACTION PLAN ⇤

1. Determine if you exhibit any signs that you lack confidence.

2. Use the Rosenberg self-esteem scale and assess your self-esteem.

3. List 3 things that you've accomplished that make you proud. _____

_____

_____

_____

4. Write down 5 of your personal strengths. _____

_____

_____

_____

_____

_____

5. Identify at least 3 situations where you've allowed others to cross your boundaries and make a plan to remedy them.

_____

_____

_____

_____

_____

6. Identify 5 confidence boosters that you will employ.

_____

_____

_____

_____

_____

7. Create or find at least 3 mantras to repeat or read every day. _____

_____

_____

_____

_____

_____

6

BUILD A WINNING ENVIRONMENT

Your environment has as much to do with who and what you are as your DNA. Create and choose it wisely.

Our physical environment—where we live, eat, sleep, play, and work—can have a tremendous impact not just on our behavior but on our chances for success. How we think and live is influenced by what and who is around us. The outcomes we are trying to achieve in life are more or less likely to happen based on the influencing conditions that we encounter daily. For example, studies have repeatedly shown that surrounding yourself with happy, successful people can increase the likelihood of you being happy and successful. Everything else being equal, putting yourself more frequently in a positive, constructive environment increases the chances that you too will be more positive and reach your goals.

When it comes specifically to weight loss, environment has a tremendous impact on what and how we eat, how we move, what we think, and our decisions to follow a plan or not. Some of these environmental influences are direct, but many others operate beneath our consciousness, which means we are not even aware of the impact they are having on our behavioral choices. We are constantly interacting with environmental forces, sometimes in conflict, at other times in harmony. There are times when we are in complete control of what comprises our environment, but there are plenty of times when we have no control at all. You might have a great plan to lose weight and transform your habits, but if the environmental conditions and your resources are not conducive to change, then success is extremely unlikely. It's important that you increase your awareness of these environmental factors that can either help or hinder your chances for success.

Let's look at some of the environmental changes you can make right away that can boost your odds of reaching your goals.

CHANGE YOUR FOOD ENVIRONMENT

One of my favorite things to tell people I coach is "You can't eat what you don't have." This is a simple statement, but the facts that underlie it are extremely consequential. Too often we set out on a path of trying to eat better and improve our health, but then we set up a minefield of temptation that's always an arm's length away. Sooner or later you're going to step on one of those mines and give in to temptation. If your plan calls for you not to eat certain foods or drink certain beverages, one of the best ways to avoid indulging in them is not to have them in your food environment at all. Out of sight doesn't always mean out of mind, but it certainly makes it much more difficult to indulge when you don't have temptation in front of you. Increase the difficulty of carrying out an action, and it's less likely you will do it.

One of the very first things you should do when starting a plan and understanding the food rules, is throw out or give away all the items in your refrigerator or cabinets that don't comply. So many people sabotage themselves by not clearing out the leftover temptations that will only become a source of constant distraction and enticement. People will often use the excuse that they don't want to waste food or money or feel bad throwing away good food when other people in the world are hungry. These sentiments are understandable, but they can also be an excuse to keep those forbidden foods and drinks around. Why would someone want to do this when they know it could result in bad decision-making and subsequent failure on their plan? One answer is that for many people, certain foods (typically high in sugar, calories, and fat) are a source of comfort. Sometimes you feel better knowing that if you're having a bad day or that craving is just too much to ignore, you can simply open the fridge or venture into a cabinet and grab that old friend that brings instant relief and satisfaction.

While throwing out the old is the first thing you should do, welcoming the new is the second. Go to the store and purchase those foods and drinks that are permissible. Put them in your kitchen, and if you have a place at work where you store snacks, put them there, too. While you might miss those chips and cookies, it will be a lot more difficult to indulge in them during your moments of weakness if they are not readily available. Controlling food presence, however, might not be so easy to do if you live with others who are not following the same eating guidelines. You can't stop a roommate from buying their favorite ice cream or a spouse from wanting to have a cupcake now and then. But you can either try finding a different place for them to store these foods or you can ask them to reduce how much of it they introduce into your shared environment.

Ian K. Smith, M.D.

WHERE YOU EAT MATTERS

Where we choose to eat can impact what and how much we eat. Studies have shown that people who eat in front of the television or computer exhibit poorer eating habits than those who actually eat at a table in a designated dining area. When you eat with distractions, you are more likely to participate in mindless eating—subconscious eating habits that can lead to unnecessary weight gain. When your attention is diverted from your food, it's easy to forget how much you've eaten. You also are not fully present with your food. You're chewing and tasting, but you're not mindful of all that the food has to offer or of your sensory reactions to the food. People who eat while doing something else also tend to choose foods that are easier to prepare or already prepackaged, and these foods tend to be less healthy. Avoid eating in your bedroom and the living room, in your car and while walking down the street. Eat in the kitchen or dining room, places where there are no digital distractions and your full attention can be given to eating and whoever is sitting at the table with you.

Avoid Situational Triggers

Knowing what triggers certain behaviors and impulses is critical to making changes that will increase your odds for success. One big universal trigger is stress. Research has consistently shown that people who are stressed often relieve this stress through eating, and this eating is rarely healthy or in appropriate quantities for someone looking to avoid consuming too many calories. Stress eating typically means consuming sweets and fat-laden foods that are full of calories and completely empty of any real nutritional value. Even the thought of eating these foods and the pleasure they bring you will begin the release of the chemical dopamine in our brains. Dopamine is an important mediator of pleasure in the brain. When an activity brings us pleasure, dopamine is released and stimulates a person to seek out even more of whatever activity caused such pleasure. In effect, dopamine reinforces pleasure, and by doing so the brain develops an expectation of experiencing the outcome that comes from a certain action. Let's say you love salty potato chips, and every time you eat them, the combination of flavor, salt, and crunch just really make you feel good. Based on dopamine and the pleasure pathway that it's part of, even just thinking about eating those chips can cause dopamine release that drives you to seek feelings of pleasure that are obtained through eating. However, these feelings of pleasure tend to be short-term and temporary, compared to the deeper, richer, longer-lasting satisfaction one might obtain from a self-generated goal.

Stress, however, is only one trigger that makes us vulnerable. Smell, sight, fatigue, and celebrations are others that you need to be mindful of avoiding or at least be prepared to handle as they relate to stimulating unhealthy decisions. Sometimes just smelling the aroma of a certain food such as the pizza dough or fresh popcorn can be a trigger that sends you off your eating plan and determinedly seeking those forbidden foods.

Extreme fatigue is another trigger for unhealthy behaviors. Sleep deprivation causes us to let our guards down and lose our inhibitions. Our focus is fuzzy, and we are more inclined to do what comes easiest and less willing to exert energy we don't seem to have to fight temptation and stick to the plan.

Getting a good night's sleep is more than just a motherly suggestion. Sleep has proven biological impact, and not getting enough of it can disrupt the body's hormonal system as well as impair judgment and decision-making.

Sleep deprivation causes impactful changes to the hormones leptin and ghrelin that regulate appetite and hunger respectively. Leptin works by suppressing appetite and encouraging the body to expend energy. When you are not getting enough sleep, the leptin levels are reduced, which means appetite increases. Ghrelin is responsible for triggering feelings of hunger. When you are sleep-deprived, ghrelin levels increase and you feel hungrier.

CREATE YOUR HAPPY SPACE

Finding a place or a driving route that makes you happy, relieved, and at peace can be a critical component for overall life balance, but particularly when it comes to traversing the sometimes arduous and winding journey of weight loss. Given all the effort required to find your motivation and keep it, execute a plan, resist temptation, and continue believing in yourself despite the obstacles you face, retreating to that special place that brings you solitude and comfort can be a game changer. You might find this place somewhere in your house or you might find it in your backyard or the woods. You might even find it in a room inside a museum. Maybe it's a certain route you take driving along a country road that makes you feel relaxed and grateful. There are no limits to where or what this happy place might be, so if you haven't already identified one, take your time and be creative in finding one. Most important, it's okay to be selfish, because this is all about you and your inner peace. It's not what others think or believe, but all about what this place or route means to you and how it makes you feel.

MODIFY YOUR WORK ENVIRONMENT

The workplace can be one of the biggest obstacles along your weight loss journey. Most work environments are not in our control, and other people have been charged with the decision-making involved in creating and maintaining it. There are all kinds of pitfalls, whether it be cafeterias with fried, greasy food, vending machines with all kinds of packaged and processed ingredients, or eating areas loaded with bins of high-calorie sweets—jobsites are often major pitfalls for those who are already barely hanging on during this tenuous journey to do better.

While there might not be much you can do about the cafeteria menu or what the vendor stocks in the machines, you can change other things to improve the food environment at your workplace.

1. Bring your own meals and snacks, whether from home or from a restaurant or café that makes them fresh.
2. Don't eat at your desk or a cafeteria that might be loaded with temptation. Find an empty office or conference room, or simply go outside. Break away from the location where you spend most of the day and enjoy the meal and conversation with a colleague.

3. Find a health buddy or small group of people who are also on a similar journey that you can eat with and even go for a walk with once or twice a day.

4. Clean out your desk to remove any foods or snacks not on your plan and fill it with those items that you are encouraged to eat.

SURROUND YOURSELF WITH PEOPLE MAKING POSITIVE DECISIONS

Who you spend most of your time with can actually make a big difference. Researchers have looked at social clusters and their interactions and have tracked corresponding behaviors and health profiles. What they found was fascinating. A thirty-two-year study published in *The New England Journal of Medicine* found the influence of having an overweight friend was stronger than if a sibling or even a spouse was obese. A Gallup poll found that 46% of overweight individuals had friends who were also overweight. This is not to suggest at all that one should not be friends with someone who is overweight. That would be ridiculous. Rather it suggests the importance of being mindful that the health decisions and behaviors exhibited by those in our close circle can enter our subconscious and influence the choices we make. Being aware of this and making a concerted effort to select the more positive influences can make a big difference.

MIT researchers found that bringing people with similar traits into a social network together with the intention of increasing physical fitness had a positive effect. Just by being in this group, more people picked up a new activity that could facilitate healthy lifestyle changes. The study went on to find that being in a network matched for common traits resulted in people being three times more likely to adopt a new health habit.

Why does this happen? One reason is a process called *mirroring*, where we tend to look at our friends to ascertain and model what is considered good or bad, as well as what's acceptable and what's not. If your inner circle spends a lot of time focusing on healthy lifestyle behaviors and making decisions that will improve health outcomes, then it is likely that you will do the same thing or at least be inspired to go in the same direction. We often try to fit in with those around us, whether it's a conscious or subconscious decision. It stands to reason that if your friends are all about living healthier, then fitting in means you will be trying to do the same thing, whether it's eating less processed food, exercising more often, or limiting your intake of foods high in calories with little nutritional value. You start leading a healthy lifestyle by the mere fact you're trying to keep up with those around you.

Friends are also good for accountability. You can confide in friends about your health struggles as well as your goals and the plan you have to reach them. Your friends can keep you accountable when you veer from the plan or exhibit behaviors that are contradictory to your mission. They can be direct and say things that others might shy away from for fear of appearing insensitive or mean-spirited. Your friends can team up with you, whether it's joining you in exercise or participating in your new style of eating. They are there to support you when things are going well and also when you've hit a rough patch and need encouragement.

Friends and social networks can also serve in a mentoring capacity. They might have experiences following a certain plan or performing certain exercise routines that are unfamiliar to you. They might possess or know of resources that can help you on your journey and give you information that can make a difference as you navigate what can be a tricky and complicated path to better health. Your friends might have already walked the steps you are now taking and can share valuable information about their experiences and help you avoid some of the mistakes they made along the way. Seek these friends out and keep them close: their wisdom can be invaluable as you work hard to stay the course and reach your goals.

You must also be wary of those who will sabotage you. The expression "Trouble loves company" is not one that should be taken lightly, for it is often the case that those who are not happy or feel deficient in some aspect will either consciously or subconsciously try to bring others down who make them feel inadequate or shine a light on their short-comings. I have heard hundreds of stories of people struggling to make a positive change in their life, only to be discouraged and sabotaged by those who are closest to them, whether it's a friend or a colleague or a spouse. At the same time, don't blame others for something you can control yourself as that is just a way of letting yourself off the hook. This might be a tough thing to do, but it's important to take a true assessment of those who truly are on your side and will support you, versus those who say they want what's best for you but are continually saying or doing things that only serve to distract you from your mission. A friend who is constantly inviting you out to eat at places that only serve food not on your plan or a spouse who continues to stock the fridge and cabinets with those forbidden treats are not part of your real support team, and you must have a direct conversation with them about this, and/or limit your exposure to them. Whether they are doing it on purpose or are simply insensitive to your struggles, the result is the same—you are being unnecessarily tempted to make decisions that will eventually cause you to deviate from your plan to achieve success.

CHANGE YOUR SOCIAL ENVIRONMENT

Many people center their social lives around activities that involve food. Whether it's celebrating a birthday at a restaurant, a catered after-hours work event, or a religious gathering—food somehow is on the agenda. And often, these foods are high in calories and lower in nutritional value. Social eating becomes an extremely permissive environment to make choices that don't conform to the plan you're following. Drinking alcohol often means overindulging in high-fat foods late at night when those extra calories will not be burned off before you go to sleep, thus creating ripe conditions for weight gain.

Celebrating an achievement shouldn't always mean that food is involved. By the same token, if there is going to be food, it doesn't always have to be the fried variety topped with fattening cream sauces or desserts laden with calories. Try going to a place where healthier options are available or when ordering from the catering menu, limit those less-healthy choices. If you're going to socialize around food, why not do it in a setting where there's also a certain amount of physical activity involved? Bowling might not be the most exertive of sports, but it's active and fun, and there is enough activity to help distract attention away from food for at least part of the time you're there.

When your friends eat those fun foods in front of you, it becomes a direct challenge to your discipline and control. Sometimes you might keep it together, but other times the temptation might be too great and you simply give in. You are only human! Reducing your exposure means reducing your vulnerability. If you know food is going to be served and the likely menu doesn't fit your plan, either eat something before you arrive at the gathering so that if you do sample some of the food you're less likely to consume a large amount, or bring a container of your own food from home.

CREATE A MOVEMENT ENVIRONMENT

When people think of exercise, they reflexively think of gyms, high-tech equipment, and trainers. But exercise comes in many forms and can be achieved in ways other than going to a fitness center. You can build a movement environment that gives you the same benefits you can achieve in a gym. Think about creative ways to add movement to your daily routine. Park in the very back of the lot that's farthest away from the door when you go to shop or to your workplace. Agree that at least twice a day you will take the steps instead of the elevator for trips that are three floors or fewer. Use wearable technology or the step counter in your smartphone to keep track of your daily steps, then after a week of creating a step log, challenge yourself the next week to increase your daily step count by 250 until you reach 10,000–12,000 per day. Find someone at work who also wants to be physically active. Meet before work to walk together or meet up during lunch for a quick fifteen-minute stroll. Take responsibility for walking the dog and be willing to go for longer distances as the weather improves. When you're on vacation, make it a point to visit local parks where you can walk and explore or even participate in some of the activities that might be offered there. When you plan social meet-ups, do so around something physically active rather than always choosing to meet over a meal.

CLEAN YOUR KITCHEN

Research has shown that messy kitchens are associated with less healthy eating habits and overindulgence. Cluttered kitchens are stressful, and stress stimulates the desire to eat "comfort" foods in many people. A messy kitchen can also be so overwhelming that a person feels like it will take too much effort to make a healthier meal or snack, so they choose a quick option that is likely prepackaged and less healthy. Kitchens that are organized influence organization in both thoughts and food preparation. This can not only influence the types of food you decide to prepare, but make cooking a pleasurable experience that you look forward to rather than dread.

⇞ ACTION PLAN ⇟

1. Create a support system.

2. List, then remove forbidden foods and temptations from your house. _____

_____

_____

_____

_____

_____

_____

3. Identify 3 triggers that encourage unhealthy decisions.

_____

_____

_____

_____

_____

_____

4. Identify your happy space. _____

_____

_____

_____

5. Change at least 2 things at work that will help you make healthier decisions. _____

_____

_____

_____

_____

6. Identify 3 positive people you can communicate with more often. _____

_____

_____

_____

7. List 3 environmental changes you will make to add more movement to your life. _____

_____

_____

_____

_____

_____

7

FIX YOUR FOOD RELATIONSHIP

Good food is more than sustenance. It's a powerful experience that should be savored and protected and never taken for granted.

Food is more than just a rich green salad full of health-boosting nutrients or a scrumptious thick dark fudge brownie with powdered sugar sprinkled on top. We eat food because our bodies need energy, but we also eat it because the actual process of eating and the flavors we taste make us feel good. We eat when we're celebrating, and we eat when we're disappointed. We eat at work functions, and we eat at the movie theater. Food is a big part of our life, an ever-present constant in interactions that involve family, business, and our social networks. We all have a unique relationship with food, and that relationship can figure heavily in our lives. Unfortunately for many people, this relationship has gone out of whack and the parameters have been stretched and pulled to the point that food has taken on an entirely different purpose than that of just sustaining and physically nourishing us. For millions of people, their relationship with food is broken, but it can be fixed.

Step one means understanding hunger and what it actually means. We don't often take much time to dissect this primal urge, but it would be wise to do so, considering the impact it can have on how and what we eat. There are two main types of hunger—physical and emotional. Physical hunger is your body's way of telling you that it needs to be nourished and you should eat something to satisfy that need. Emotional hunger is your mind telling you that you need to eat a specific thing to make yourself feel better or distracted from something that might be troubling you. Sometimes it's not always clear which hunger you're experiencing, but being able to distinguish between the two can go a long way toward helping you fix the problem.

EMOTIONAL EATING

Through research and vast treatment experience, experts have done a great job at identifying and describing some of the common signs that might indicate that a person has a penchant for emotional eating. There is no magic number of how many of these signs you need to experience in order to be considered an emotional eater, but it's very likely that if one on the list applies to you, there's probably at least one or two others that also match your relationship with food. Read the following list and see if any apply to you, and if so, how many?

1. **YOU EAT WHEN YOU'RE NOT HUNGRY.** Normal physiological functioning cues eating to satisfy hunger. Your body is wired so that when it is in need of calories (energy) or nourishment, it lets you know that it needs to be fed. But if you find yourself

reaching for food even when you're not hungry, but rather when you're feeling lonely, angry, stressed, or sad, this can be a sign that you're an emotional eater.

2. **YOU FEEL GUILTY FOR EATING.** You are about to take a big bite of a chocolate cupcake with buttercream frosting. And while the saliva is building inside your mouth you think, "I know I'm not supposed to be eating this, but . . ." You eat the cupcake, but when you're done, you are shouldered with heavy guilt for doing so. You knew you weren't supposed to eat it, but you ate it anyway. You enjoyed eating it. Then you feel guilty. It's a pattern you repeat often. The guilt you already know you're going to experience never stops you from going through with the behavior.

3. **YOU EAT IMPULSIVELY.** You don't think too much before eating. You simply go and purchase things that look good to you that you know will make you feel good. Maybe you just feel the urge to open up that favorite snacks drawer and pull out whatever's in there, even if you're not physically hungry. Impulsive eaters quickly grab what they can and give very little

thought to the pros and cons of doing so and are often unable to stop until they have overeaten.

4. **YOU EAT TO FEEL HAPPY.** Sure, really delicious food will make you feel good when you're eating it. There's nothing wrong with being happy when you eat tasty food. But when you eat food for the sole purpose of improving your mood and getting an emotional lift, this can be concerning. When food becomes one of your main sources of happiness, then red flags should start flapping in your mind. Food is no longer sustenance or a culinary adventure for you; rather, it is a treatment, like a prescription medication or counseling sessions with a therapist.

5. **YOU HIDE WHAT YOU'RE EATING FROM OTHERS.** You either rarely eat in front of others, or when you do, you barely eat at all. Then when you're alone, you eat the way you really want to indulge without inhibitions. This likely happens because you are embarrassed to let someone see what and how you eat, because you're worried they'll think less of you or finally discover your unhealthy relationship

EMOTIONAL HUNGER	PHYSICAL HUNGER
You have cravings for only certain foods	You desire a diverse group of foods
Comes on suddenly without warning	Develops gradually over time
Difficult to satisfy, so you eat until you're uncomfortably full, and even then you might not feel satisfied	Easy to feel satisfied with a normal quantity of food
Might trigger feelings of guilt, shame, or regret	You don't feel bad about yourself or have any negative feelings about eating
Felt mostly in your thoughts without a physical component	Physically feel hunger pangs within your stomach

with food. You might also be hiding your eating, because you know it's unhealthy or not part of your program, so the last thing you want is the annoyance of someone confirming what you already know.

6. **YOU EAT WHEN YOU'RE STRESSED.** When you are feeling stressed and anxious about some-

thing, the first thing you reach for is that bag of potato chips or carton of ice cream. Food has become your go-to answer when you're feeling pressured or worried and life just seems to be overwhelming you and you need a release. Eating takes your mind off your problems and calms you. It's like a good sedative: reliable, effective, and relatively inexpensive.

7. **YOU FIND COMFORT IN FOOD.** Food becomes a coping mechanism that you turn to time and time again. Eating isn't just an experience of physical satisfaction, but one of emotional satisfaction as well. You are away from friends and family for an extended period of time—you find comfort in eating. You are disappointed in a romantic relationship—you turn to food. Work is troubling you—food is your answer. There's a reason why they call it comfort food, and you take that to the next level.

8. **YOU FEEL LIKE YOUR EATING IS OUT OF CONTROL, BUT YOU'RE POWERLESS TO STOP EATING.** You open a bag of chocolate chip cookies and your intention is to have only a couple of them.

Fifteen minutes later you find yourself scooping up crumbs at the bottom of a now empty bag. You had told yourself that you were going to enjoy just a few, be satisfied, and put the rest away for another time. In fact, you might have even put the bag back in the cabinet. But after a few minutes you pulled the bag back out and commenced popping more cookies into your mouth.

9. **YOU REWARD YOURSELF WITH FOOD.** You have a good day at work and your boss commends you on your presentation. You celebrate by stopping by the ice-cream parlor and loading up on a chocolate sundae. You finish a tedious home project after months of struggling to get it done. You rip open a big bag of salt-and-vinegar popcorn. You turn to food not just when you're hungry, but as a reward for a job well done. Food has become your equivalent of a victory lap: instead of running around the stadium to the cheers of the crowd, you visit the grocery store or bakery and load up on fat and sugar. Your celebrations almost always involve food, and other rewards pale in comparison.

10. **FOOD KEEPS YOU COMPANY.** It's not easy feeling lonely or like no one really understands you. Food becomes an instant companion and, in many respects, the perfect one. It doesn't talk back to you. You can have it when you want and then put it away when it's served its purpose. It's with you while you're watching TV and never complains about watching the same episode for the tenth time. Food has become a "friend." You aren't putting that frozen pizza in the microwave because you're hungry, but because it's something to do and you feel happier and more fulfilled eating it.

CHECK YOUR EMOTIONAL EATING

Not all emotional eaters suffer equally or have the same type or number of issues that need to be addressed. Your signs and symptoms might be mild, or they might be severe. Professional counseling can help you make this determination. But even without the help of an expert, there are things you can do to help get yourself back on track, achieve better self-awareness, and make important behavioral changes. Try some or all of the following activities, as they can make a real difference in how you respond when faced with emotional and situational triggers.

1. **KEEP A FOOD JOURNAL.** Sometimes writing down what you're eating can also keep you better attuned to your areas of strengths and weaknesses. This can also serve as a deterrent from unhealthy food choices or eating behaviors. The simple act of documenting what you do leads to accountability. Most of us have an inner drive to do well and "bring home a good report card." Keeping your own score along the way can become a great motivator to change or modify your eating behaviors and patterns.

2. **DO A HUNGER CHECK.** Before eating, ask yourself if you're really hungry. This might sound simple and obvious, but think about the last time you questioned yourself before digging in. You probably don't remember. On a hunger scale of 0 to 10, with 0 meaning you're completely satiated and 10 meaning you're ravenously hungry, rate your hunger

first. Eat when you are in the 3 to 4 range. Avoid the extremes near 0 and above 8, as you will either be eating when you're not hungry or waiting until your hunger is overpowering and you're more likely to overindulge or make poor choices.

3. **AVOID BOREDOM.** When people are bored, they tend to make decisions without giving them much discerning thought. This is particularly true when it comes to food consumption. Some people turn to food when they're bored, not because they're hungry, rather eating becomes just another thing that can be done to fill the time. Instead, stay active. Find other activities like reading, writing, or exercising that keep you engaged, and eat only when your body truly needs to be nourished.

4. **REMOVE TEMPTATION.** You're less likely to be tempted by foods or beverages you can't see or smell, instead of those staring right at you, just begging for you to consume. Keeping a bowl of candy on your desk or frozen pizza next to the frozen fruit is only going to get that dopamine wave rushing through your

brain, and before you know it, the wrapper is off and you're satisfying that gnawing craving. Out of sight might not always be out of mind, but it's a lot better than when the tempting food is right under your nose.

5. **EAT WITH OTHERS.** When you share a meal with others, it's more likely that you will be able to keep your impulses in check. Barring the pizza party or late-night bar crawl, it's more typically the case that when you sit down with friends and other loved ones to eat, you want to stay in control. Eating with others can have a positive effect on your own food choices. You most likely won't order the cheeseburger and fries when everyone else is having salad and fish. (But if you're not careful, the choices your dining partners make can have a negative influence and prompt you to eat those foods you are trying to avoid.) Having company while eating also means having conversation. This means you will eat slowly, rather than rushing through the meal. Eating too fast can lead to overeating because you're not giving your stomach enough time to communicate with

your brain that you're full. Slow down to savor the meal and enjoy the company.

6. **HAVE MORE FUN.** It's as simple as it sounds. When you feel that urge to eat and you know it's not from hunger, do something like take a walk in your neighborhood with someone and have a nice conversation. Organize old photos from past vacations. Find a fun way to be distracted from whatever emotion or situation that is triggering you to eat. Play with an animal or read an interesting book. The more time you spend happy and having fun, the less time available for you to be sad or emotionally vulnerable. When you're having fun, food is pushed to the back of your mind and your current activity keeps you fully engaged.

7. **RELIEVE YOUR STRESS IN OTHER WAYS.** Do something like watch a movie or TV show that engages your mind so that you're not thinking about what is stressing you. Listen to music, read a book, occupy your hands with a small craft project, call a friend and talk on the phone, or take a warm bath

or shower. Find things that will focus your attention elsewhere and comfort you at the same time.

8. **EAT SOMETHING HEALTHY.** When you eat healthier foods that physically satisfy you, it can be easier to recognize when you're eating just to satisfy an emotional yearning. Healthier snacks such as vegetables with hummus, fresh fruit, nuts, and un-buttered popcorn seasoned with a modest amount of salt are great options to help control the extent and impact of emotional eating.

9. **DO SOMETHING PHYSICAL.** Exercising can release endorphins, the body's happy chemicals that can make you feel good and energized. If you're feel-ing a little down or uninterested or overwhelmed with thoughts that are racing through your mind, doing something physical can be not only a great dis-traction but a positive way to help you reach some of your weight loss goals.

10. **PRACTICE MINDFUL EATING.** This type of eating develops awareness of your eating habits, giv-

ing you an important opportunity to hit the pause button between triggers and your reaction to them. The goal is to focus your full attention around your cravings as well as your physical cues and sensory experience while eating. Take time to enjoy the taste of the food and try to discern the different ingredients and what they add to the overall experience. Allow your senses to be fully engaged beyond the taste alone. Appreciate the smells, sounds, colors, and textures of the food you are eating.

11. **GET SUPPORT.** Call someone to have a conversation about what's troubling you. Lean on family or friends to support you and help you stay on track. There are plenty of support groups you can join, whether in person or online. Just having someone who will listen to you and share their experiences can be tremendously helpful when you're struggling and feel like you're in it alone.

There are several situations and emotions that can cause emotional eating. It's important that you try to identify your triggers. Awareness of those triggers can be the first step in overcoming your emotional ties to food that cause you to eat in an unhealthy manner. Ask yourself if any of the following situations or emotions prompt you to eat rather than using another coping strategy.

⟫ **EMOTIONAL/SITUATIONAL TRIGGERS** ⟪

+ Stress
+ Depression
+ Anger
+ Boredom
+ Sadness/depression
+ Anxiety
+ Loneliness
+ Difficult change
+ Feelings of low self-worth
+ Frustration
+ Fight with a friend or loved one
+ Trying to fit in with others
+ Fear of missing out

FOOD ADDICTION

For a long time, the concept of food addiction was derided and scoffed at by professionals in the field. Many called it a fake diagnosis, while others called it nothing more than an excuse people used to explain away their greed and inability to maintain control. To say that the concept of food addiction has been controversial is an understatement. There is a school of thought where leaders think that real addictions are limited to psychoactive substances that produce clear, defined symptoms such as physical tolerance, dependence, and withdrawal. And there is the other school of thought that acknowledges that food can be the object of an addiction just like a drug or gambling or excessive shopping.

What really got scientists to start changing their opinions and their approach to people who couldn't control their eating impulses came from the similarities to substance addiction. They found that there was significant overlap in the symptoms, risk factors, and neurobiological characteristics between well-studied substance addiction and what was starting to emerge as food addiction. As with other addictions, neurotransmitters (chemical messengers within the brain) and their interaction with the brain's reward system have been also associated with food addiction. These addictive behaviors and conditions include intense impulses to eat certain foods, the inability to resist these impulses or cravings, extreme satisfaction associated with eating, and the dependence one develops on food to satisfy both physical and emotional needs.

When it was believed that people who overindulged suffered from some type of vulnerability, treatment centered around interventional therapies that focused on a person's interaction with others as well as their food environment. But with the growing belief that there is a neurobiological underpinning to food addiction, a new cadre of treatment options became available for therapists who began seeing more patients exhibiting symptoms of food addiction.

How do you know if you suffer from food addiction? This diagnosis is not always clear cut, and experts haven't yet nailed down what specific behaviors you must exhibit to fall into this category of eating disorders. Plenty of research, however, has been conducted over the years to give experts a very good sense of common symptoms shared by food addicts. You can still have a food addiction even if all the symptoms don't apply to you. These are some general guidelines that can at least give you an idea if food addiction is a possibility and prompt you to seek treatment.

⤞ **SYMPTOMS OF FOOD ADDICTION** ⤝

1. Eating to the point of physical pain or discomfort
2. Obsessive food cravings
3. Experiencing cravings despite being full and not hungry
4. Eating much more than you intended to eat
5. Your thoughts are constantly preoccupied with obtaining and eating food
6. Rationalizing why you should eat a food that you know you shouldn't be eating
7. Your eating negatively impacts social interactions, finances, and/or family life

---

8. Feelings of guilt after eating, but still doing it again soon
9. Continual binge eating
10. Continued relapses where you fail to follow rules you set for yourself to control eating

MANAGING AND OVERCOMING FOOD ADDICTION

Entire books and lengthy research papers have been written on this topic. There is no one solution that works for everyone, and sometimes solving an addiction requires a multifaceted approach. There are plenty of counselors and addiction specialists who have had vast experience helping people who have a pathological relationship with food. The answers to this problem can be as complicated as the problem itself. It might take several attempts using different approaches for you to find success, but be encouraged that success is very possible and many have overcome their addiction to food and never looked back.

The foundation for any successful intervention needs to be centered on your awareness of the intricacies of and connections within your addiction. The first thing you need to understand is the underlying basis for your relationship with food. There are some basic questions that only you can answer, but these answers are pivotal to how you will move forward to find solutions.

1. What situations and emotions trigger you to eat when you're not physically hungry?
2. Do you believe you have an inappropriate relationship with food? If yes, what makes you think so? If not, why not?
3. How does eating the foods you crave make you feel while you're eating? How do you feel afterward?
4. What situations make you think about eating?
5. Is your concern for your weight truly connected to your eating habits?
6. What environments spark your unhealthy eating and/or exercise habits?
7. What has stopped you from eating and exercising better?

Once you've answered these questions, you can start focusing on some of your trouble areas. Trying to avoid your triggers is the first thing you might try, but sometimes triggers are unavoidable; look to modify the length and type of your interaction with the exposure. For example: your boss is constantly giving you a hard time and you're having daily confrontations, but unfortunately there's no way to avoid your boss since you have to go to work. Try reducing how often you interface with your boss, and when you must interact, change the dynamic by taking a more positive approach and signaling that you're not willing to engage in negativity. For example, if a conversation you're having veers into territory that you find uncomfortable or disagreeable, steer it in another direction with a smile on your face and nonconfrontational tone.

THE GOLDILOCKS PRINCIPLE

In the fairy tale "Goldilocks and the Three Bears," the little girl Goldilocks enters the unoccupied house of the three bears and discovers three bowls of porridge on the kitchen table. She tries the first one, but it's too hot. She tries the second one, but it's too cold. But the third one is just the right temperature, so she happily eats it all. Finding the right balance in what and how we eat as well as our relationship with food is critical. There is no *one* way that's the right way, and we all have to find what works for us by trying different strategies and methods. In fact, there may even be different ways for each person depending on the time of the day or day of the week or where they might be in their life. No one can or should eat perfectly all the time, so finding that right mix of healthy and "fun" foods is important to avoid feeling deprived and frustrated. Take your time finding that bowl of porridge!

AWARENESS MAKES YOU PRESENT

By keeping in touch with your body and your emotions and what food means to you, you will have better control over your impulses and eating behaviors. Even if an emotional trigger leads you to the refrigerator, all is not lost if you pull out something healthy rather than last night's fried leftovers drenched in a cream sauce. It's your awareness of your individual strengths and weaknesses that will serve as the backbone for developing a healthy relationship with food or fixing a food relationship that has been broken. It requires an open mind, patience, and a belief that eventually you will find the right fit, and that fit will make you happy. Eating great, tasty food should be an experience enjoyed and not one that makes you feel guilty or embarrassed. At the end of the day, the rule of moderation is still the cord that can tether us to a food life that is well lived and positive, a vital part of who we are.

⇗ ACTION PLAN ⇖

1. Determine if you use food for something other than sustenance.

2. List 3 ways you plan to make sure you're responding to physical hunger versus emotional hunger. _____

_____

_____

_____

_____

_____

_____

3. List any emotional or situational triggers that prompt you to eat. _____

_____

_____

_____

_____

_____

4. Practice doing a hunger check before eating.

5. Think of a fun project you can undertake and resort to when starting to feel bored. _____

_____

_____

_____

6. Review the symptoms of food addiction and determine if you experience any of them. If so, choose at least 3 strategies to help you manage or overcome them.

_____

_____

_____

_____

_____

_____

7. Time how long it takes for you to eat a sit-down meal and aim for a total time of at least 30 minutes.

FINAL THOUGHTS

No one has ever been perfect. That is a record that will never be broken, so don't waste good energy chasing an unreachable dream. But you can still be really good and extremely happy if you put your mind to it and believe above all else that your goals are realistic and possible, and you have what it takes to achieve them. The journey of losing and maintaining a healthy weight is as long and unpredictable, as tortured and thrilling, as the journey of life itself. With the right mental approach and outlook, you can find enormous success and happiness, but it really starts with what springs from your own mind and how you nourish and cultivate that sprout.

A critical component in setting and reaching goals is understanding who and what you are and who you want to be. The beauty of our uniqueness is that we each have a mind that allows us to dream and imagine and create the life we want to live and the people we want to be. Finding meaningful success in life means having a willingness to acknowledge and improve on your weaknesses as well as recognizing and enhancing your strengths. Finding success on a weight loss plan starts with having an honest conversation with yourself about heightening your self-awareness and understanding who you are. When you start from a place of truth and self-reflection, then you can develop an honest and realistic vision of what you want to accomplish and the best way to get there.

Weight loss is difficult, for some more than others. It is frustrating and at times elusive, often rewarding and at times humiliating. It doesn't always happen when it's supposed to happen, and often it doesn't meet the expectations we have of it. But if you develop a love for yourself and a healthy relationship with food and movement, and you adopt sound guiding principles that teach you how to make better choices, weight loss can be manageable and even enjoyable as you transform into your best you. Love yourself with all your imperfections. Remain determined even in the face of hardship. Never be afraid to let your mind dream regardless of how far away the dreams feel from your reality. Almost every day I drive by a simple metal sign posted on the side of the road with no brand logo or advertising pitch on it. Rather just three simple words that you should repeat often and never forget: YOU ARE BEAUTIFUL.

To find a plan that might work for you, check out my app Dr. Ian's World. Go to www.DrIansWorld.com

MIND OVER WEIGHT
TOP 10 THOUGHTS
TO LIVE BY

1. Every day is a chance to hit the reset button.
2. Find comfort in your strengths and consider weaknesses your opportunities.
3. It's not always about hitting your goals; instead, it's about the effort you put into reaching them.
4. A clear vision can declutter a busy mind.
5. Motivation gets you started, and commitment keeps you going.
6. Positive energy breeds positive results.
7. Focus not on how far away from a goal you are, but on how far you've come.

8. Failure is an opportunity to improve.
9. The only comparison that matters is in your mirror.
10. Your mind is like a muscle: the more you exercise it, the stronger it becomes.

INDEX

Index

Index

Index